Sanitation and Cleanliness for a Healthy Environment

by Jeff Conant and Pam Fadem

This book is part of a larger volume, *A Community Guide to Environmental Health.*

Copyright © 2008, 2015 by Hesperian Health Guides

Sanitation and Cleanliness   ISBN 978-0-942364-57-6

A Community Guide to Environmental Health   ISBN 978-0-942364-56-9

Contact us:

Hesperian Health Guides
2860 Telegraph Ave.
Oakland, California, 94609 USA
tel: 510-845-1447
email: *hesperian@hesperian.org*
website: *www.hesperian.org*

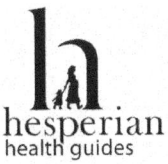

hesperian
health guides

Sanitation and Cleanliness for a Healthy Environment

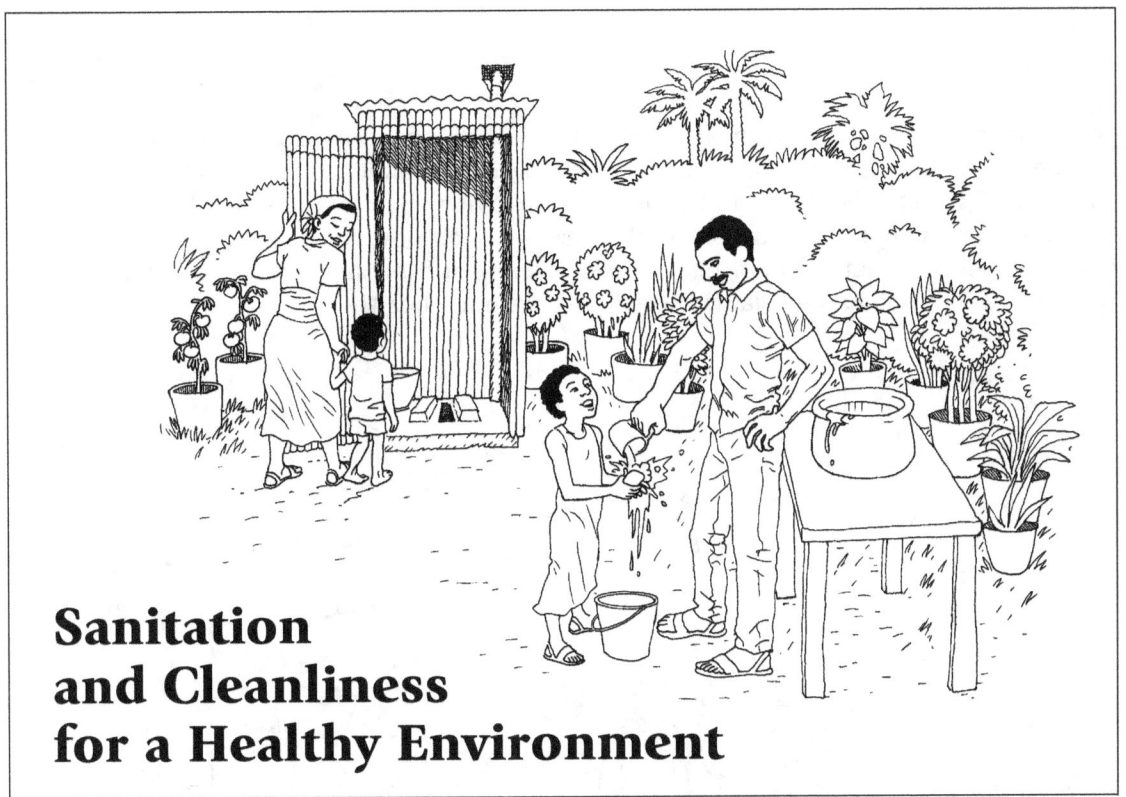

Sanitation and Cleanliness for a Healthy Environment

Human waste (feces and urine) can pollute water, food, and soil leading to serious health problems, such as diarrhea, worms, cholera, and bladder infections. Good health can be promoted and many of these problems can be prevented through:

- personal cleanliness (*hygiene*) — washing hands, bathing, and wearing clean clothes.
- public cleanliness (*sanitation*) — building and using clean and safe toilets, keeping water sources clean, and disposing of garbage safely.

All of the toilets described in this booklet will dispose of human waste so it does not contaminate our drinking water, food, or hands. Some of the toilets have the added benefit of turning dangerous waste into fertilizer for farmers to use on their fields or fruit trees. This is called *ecological* sanitation.

Just as important as a safe and comfortable toilet is a way to wash hands after using it. Safe toilets and hand-washing can prevent most of the illnesses that come from germs in human waste.

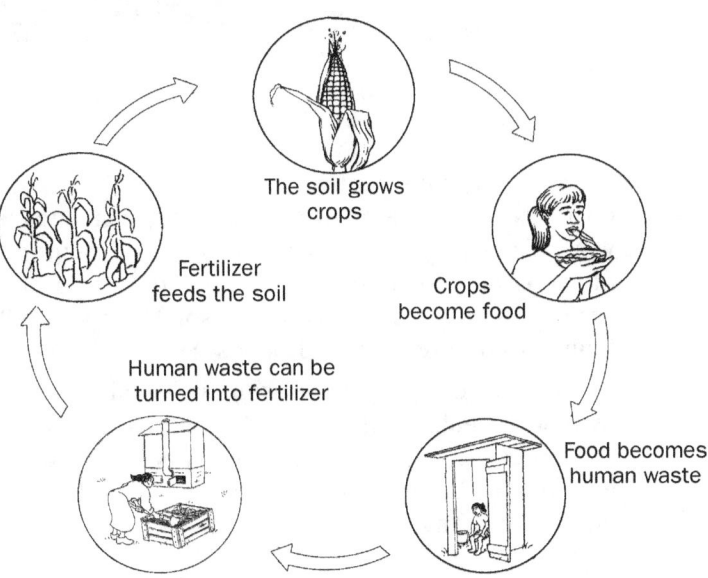

The soil grows crops

Fertilizer feeds the soil

Human waste can be turned into fertilizer

Crops become food

Food becomes human waste

Ecological sanitation turns waste into a resource.

Promoting sanitation

Some health workers believe health problems and death from poor sanitation can be prevented only if people change their personal habits, or change their "behaviors" for staying clean. But promoting behavior change often fails because the conditions people face in their daily lives, such as poverty or lack of clean water, or decent toilets, do not change. And when their behavior does not change, the people themselves are blamed for their own poor health.

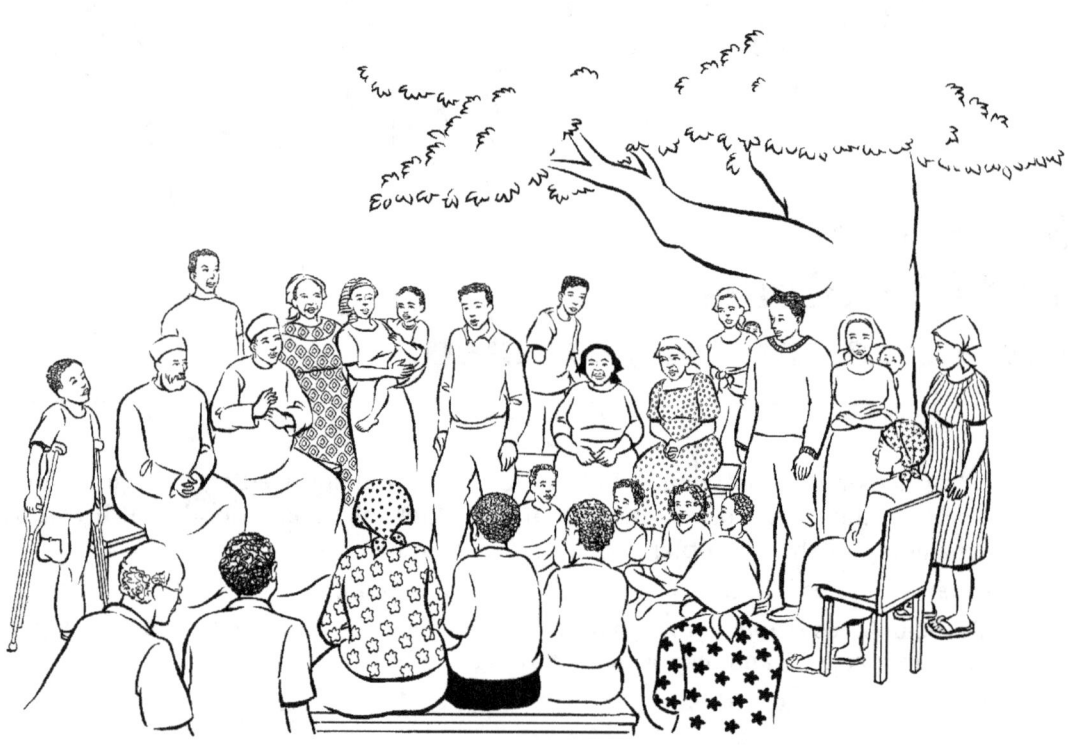

Experts may offer technical solutions, such as modern toilets that use no water, or costly sewage treatment systems. But just because these technical solutions may work elsewhere does not mean they will respond to the traditions or conditions of the community. Some of the toilets in this booklet may not be right for some communities. Offering technical solutions without understanding peoples' cultures, living conditions and real needs can create more problems than it solves.

Diseases caused by poor sanitation will continue if people are blamed for their own poor health or if technical solutions that ignore local conditions are promoted. To improve health in a lasting way, health promoters must listen carefully and work with people in the community to develop solutions based on their needs, abilities, and desire for change.

What people want from toilets

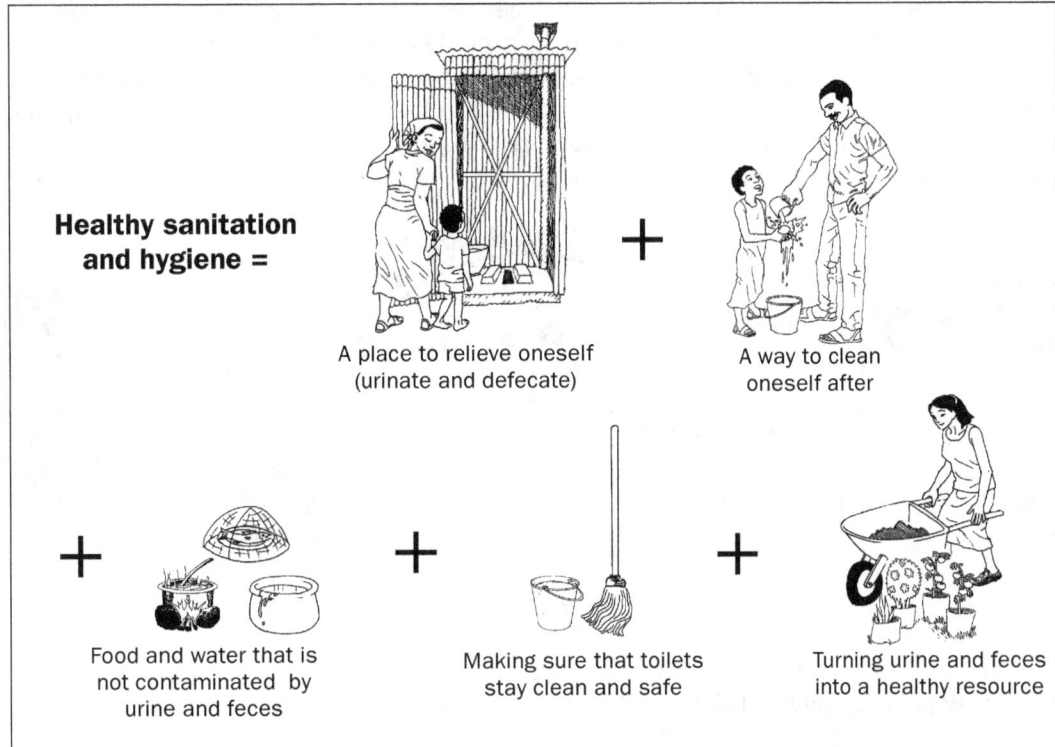

Healthy sanitation and hygiene =

A place to relieve oneself (urinate and defecate)

+

A way to clean oneself after

+

Food and water that is not contaminated by urine and feces

+

Making sure that toilets stay clean and safe

+

Turning urine and feces into a healthy resource

Health is not always the main reason why people want improved sanitation. People also want:

Privacy: A toilet can be as simple as a deep hole in the ground. But the need for privacy makes it important for a toilet to have a good shelter with a door. The best shelters are simple and are built from local materials.

Safety: For a toilet to be safe it must be well-built and in a safe place. If a toilet is badly built it can be dangerous to use. And if the toilet is far from the home or in an isolated place, women may be in danger of sexual violence when they use it.

Comfort: People will more likely use a toilet with a comfortable place to sit or squat, and a shelter large enough to stand up in. They will also be more likely to use a toilet that is close to the house and that is sheltered from wind, rain, or snow.

Cleanliness: If a toilet is dirty and smelly, no one will want to use it. Traditionally, cleaning toilets is the job of women and low-status people. If cleaning toilets becomes a shared responsibility in the community, it is more likely they will be properly used and cared for.

Respect: A well-kept toilet brings status and respect to its owner. Often this is a very important reason for people to spend the money and effort to build one.

Safe water for washing and drinking is also important for health. So are other kinds of cleanliness such as ensuring that women have a way to keep clean during monthly bleeding. (For more about how women are hurt by poor sanitation, see pages 21 to 22.)

How does poor sanitation lead to health problems?

Illnesses caused by germs and worms in feces are a constant source of discomfort for millions of people. Infections caused by roundworms, whipworms, pinworms, hookworms, and blood flukes (shistosomiasis) can cause many types of diarrhea diseases such as dysentery, typhoid, giardia and cholera. These can spread rapidly, leading to dehydration, anemia, and malnutrition, and cholera can bring a rapid death to many people. The illnesses caused by these infections share many signs:

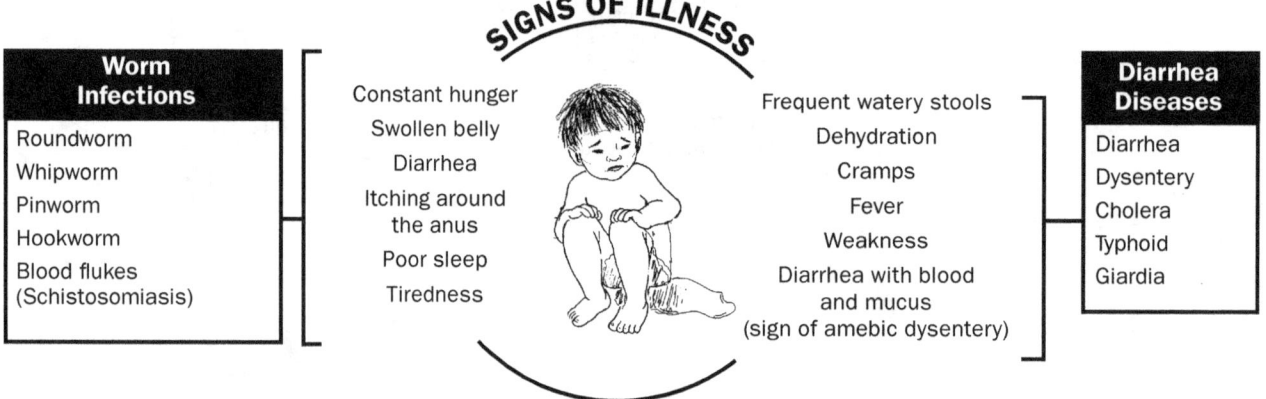

SIGNS OF ILLNESS

Worm Infections		Diarrhea Diseases
Roundworm	Constant hunger	Frequent watery stools
Whipworm	Swollen belly	Dehydration
Pinworm	Diarrhea	Cramps
Hookworm	Itching around the anus	Fever
Blood flukes (Schistosomiasis)	Poor sleep	Weakness
	Tiredness	Diarrhea with blood and mucus (sign of amebic dysentery)

Worm Infections: Roundworm, Whipworm, Pinworm, Hookworm, Blood flukes (Schistosomiasis)

Diarrhea Diseases: Diarrhea, Dysentery, Cholera, Typhoid, Giardia

To learn more about treating diarrhea diseases and worm infections, see Chapters 12 and 13 (especially pages 131 to 161) in the book *Where There is No Doctor.*

How germs spread disease

Many illnesses are spread from person to person by germs. Germs are tiny living things that cause sickness. Sometimes it is easy to know where germs are — in feces, rotting foods, and other dirty places. But sometimes, germs are in places that look and smell clean. Germs can pass directly from person to person through touch, and sometimes through the air with dust or when people cough or sneeze. If these germs get in food or water, they can cause diarrhea when we eat or drink.

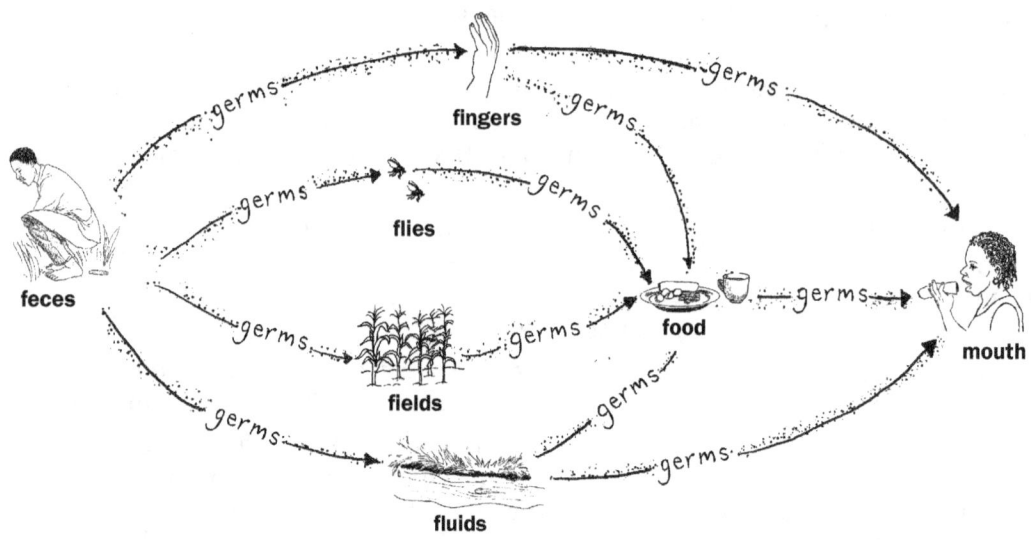

Sometimes it is easier to remember the ways germs travel by showing that they are all words beginning with the letter "F": fingers, flies, fields, foods, and fluids (water).

Here is one way that germs spread disease:

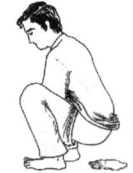
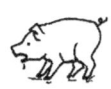
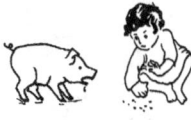
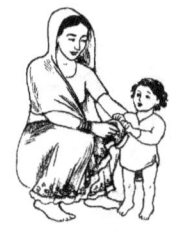

1. A man has diarrhea outside.

2. A pig eats the man's feces.

3. A child plays with the pig and gets feces on his hands.

4. The child starts to cry and his mother comforts him. He wipes his hands on her skirt.

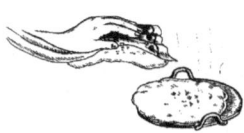
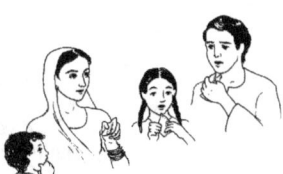
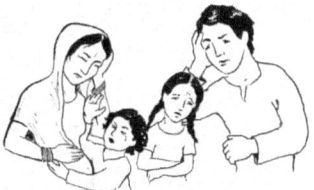

5. The mother cooks for the family. She uses her soiled skirt to keep from burning her hands. The feces from her skirt gets on her hands. She serves the food.

6. The family eats the food.

7. Later, the whole family has diarrhea.

What could have prevented the family's illness?

The spread of illness could have been prevented:

- if the man had used a toilet.
- if the pig was kept in a fenced area.
- if the child had washed his hands, rather than used his mother's skirt.
- if the mother had not touched her soiled skirt and then touched the food.
- if the mother had washed her hands with soap and water.

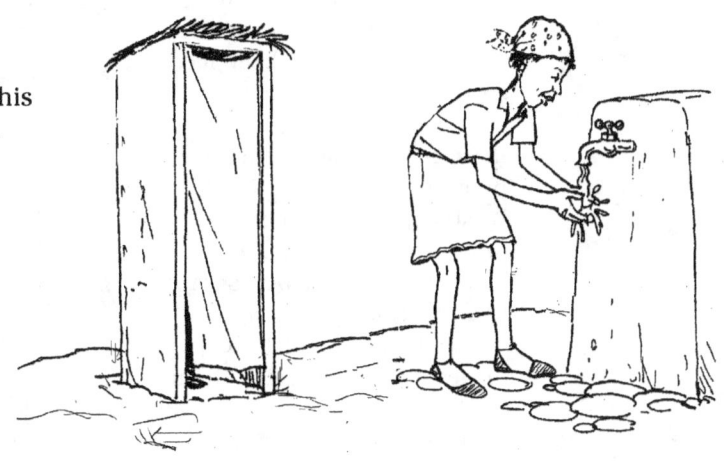

Here are some ways to prevent the spread of germs and worms:

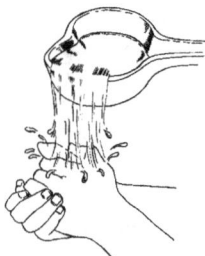

Wash hands

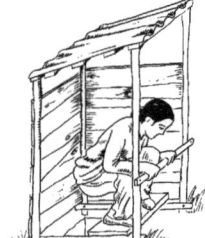

Use a toilet

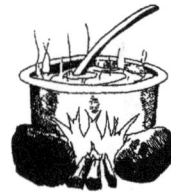

Cook food

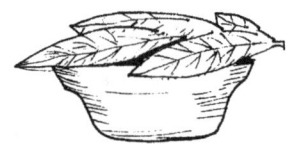

Cover food

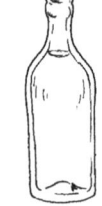

Protect and disinfect water

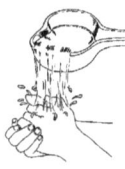

Always wash hands before and after using the toilet and before handling food. Use clean water and soap if available. If not, use clean sand or ash.

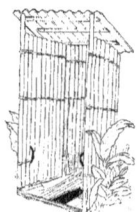

Use a toilet. This puts germs and worms out of contact with people. If there is no toilet it is best to defecate far from sources of water, in a place where feces will not be touched by people or animals. Cover it with dirt to keep flies away.

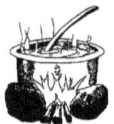

Use clean and safe methods of preparing and storing food. Wash fruits and vegetables or cook them well before eating them. Feed food scraps to animals or put them in a compost pile or toilet. Keep dishes clean after using them.

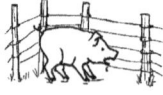

Keep animals away from household food and community water sources.

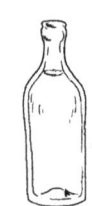

Protect water sources and use clean water for drinking and washing.

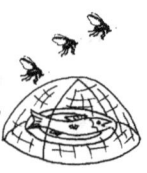

Make fly-traps and cover food. This can prevent flies from spreading germs. Toilets that control flies or stop them from breeding can help (see page 32 and pages 37 to 41).

A fly-trap made of a plastic bottle

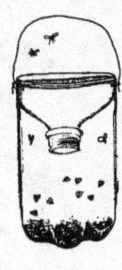

1. Cut the top part off a plastic bottle.
2. Attach wire or string to the bottle for hanging.
3. Put some sweet bait, like sugar or fruit, in the bottle.
4. Put the top back in the bottle upside-down.
5. Flies will fly in but will not be able to fly out.
6. When the bottle is full, empty it into a toilet or compost pile.

Bladder and kidney infections

Infections of the bladder and kidney are caused by germs. These infections are much more common in women than in men because germs can easily get into the body through the urinary opening near the vagina. Infections of the urinary system can be mild or severe and even life-threatening.

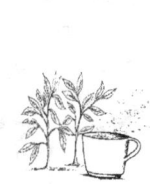

Causes of bladder infections

Germs can enter the urinary opening and cause infection when a woman:

A girl or woman of any age — even a small baby — can get an infection of her urine system.

- goes a long time without urinating. Try to urinate every 3 or 4 hours.

- goes a long time without drinking liquids. Try to drink at least 8 glasses or cups of clean water a day. Drink even more when working in the hot sun.

- does not keep her genitals clean. Try to wash the genitals every day, and always wipe from front to back after using the toilet.

- has sex. This is one of the most common causes of bladder infection in women. To prevent infection, urinate after having sex. This washes the germs that cause bladder infections out of the urine tube.

Signs and treatment

Signs of bladder or urinary tract infection include:

- Need to urinate often and urgently
- Pain in the lower belly just after urinating
- Burning feeling when urinating
- Urinating without control
- Reddish or cloudy urine
- Foul-smelling urine

If you have signs of a bladder infection, start drinking plenty of water to help flush out germs. If a bladder infection goes untreated, it can worsen and infect your kidneys. If the signs last more than 2 days, you may need medicines.

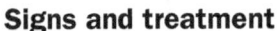

Signs of kidney infection include:

- Any bladder infection signs
- Pain in the lower back
- Fever and chills
- Nausea and vomiting
- Diarrhea
- Feeling very weak and ill

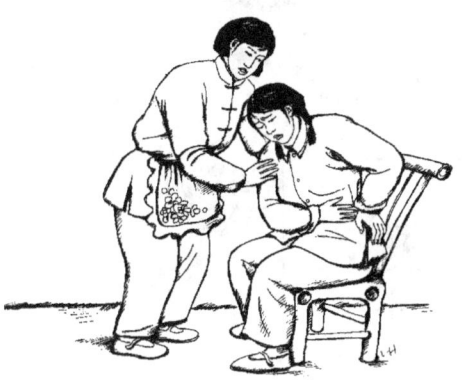

Kidney infections are more serious than bladder infections because the kidney can get so sick that it stops working. While plenty of water, herbal remedies, or sulfa drugs usually cure a urinary tract infection, a kidney infection often needs more treatment. If you have the signs of a kidney infection, see a health worker right away.

To learn more about treating bladder and kidney infections, see the book *Where Women Have No Doctor*, pages 366 to 368.

Diarrhea and dehydration

Many people die from diarrhea diseases, especially children. These diseases are often caused when germs get into drinking water or food. Most children who die from diarrhea die because they do not have enough water left in their bodies. This lack of water is called dehydration.

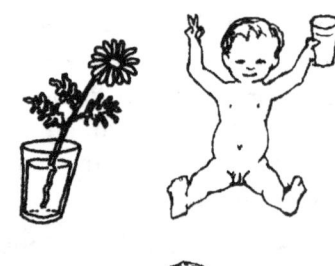

People of any age can become dehydrated, but dehydration can happen very quickly to small children and is most dangerous for them.

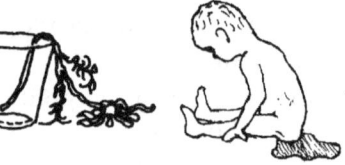

Any child with watery diarrhea is in danger of dehydration.

Signs of dehydration

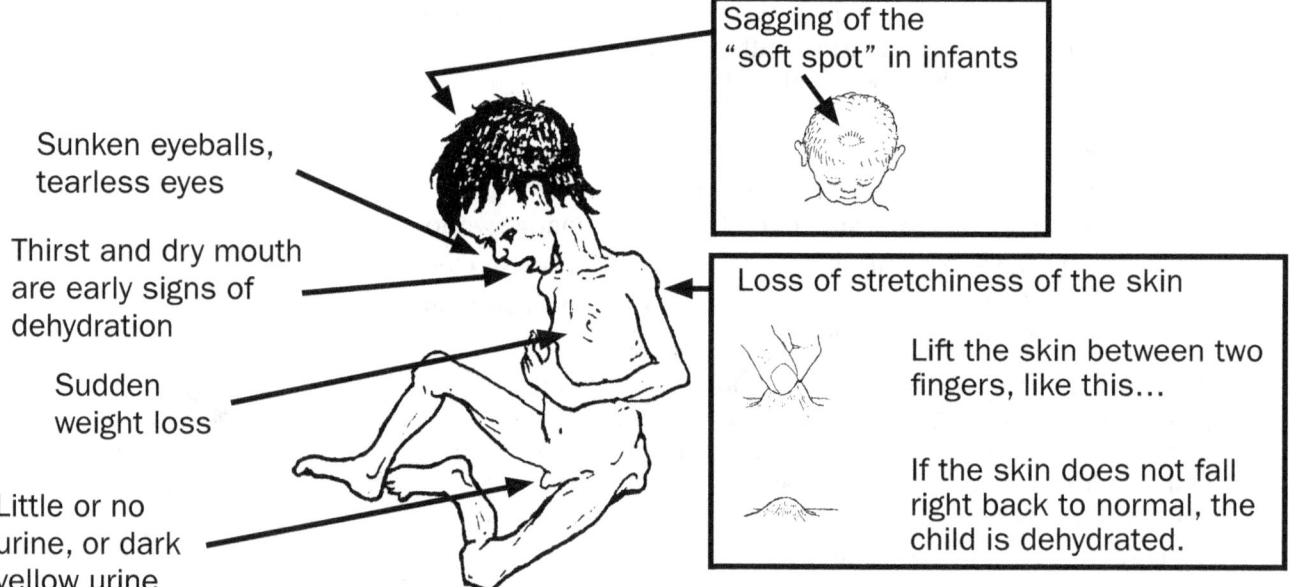

Sagging of the "soft spot" in infants

Sunken eyeballs, tearless eyes

Thirst and dry mouth are early signs of dehydration

Sudden weight loss

Little or no urine, or dark yellow urine

Loss of stretchiness of the skin

Lift the skin between two fingers, like this...

If the skin does not fall right back to normal, the child is dehydrated.

Note for the health worker _____

To teach the signs of dehydration, you can use a "body mapping" activity. Bring parents together and show them a picture of a healthy baby. Have them point or draw arrows to where they would see signs of dehydration. Discuss all the signs. Then discuss the ways they can help their children when these signs appear — and what they can do to prevent dehydration and diarrhea in the first place.

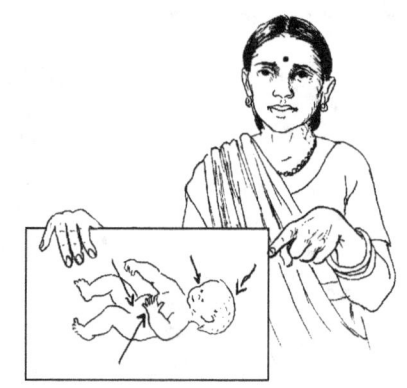

To stop dehydration

When a child has watery diarrhea or diarrhea and vomiting, do not wait for signs of dehydration. Act quickly.

Give lots of liquids to drink, such as a thin cereal porridge or gruel, soup, water, or rehydration drink (see below).

Keep giving food. As soon as the sick child (or adult) can eat food, give frequent feedings of foods he likes. To babies, keep giving breast milk often – and before other drinks.

Rehydration drink helps to prevent or to treat dehydration. It does **not** cure diarrhea, but may give enough time for the diarrhea to cure itself.

Rehydration drink

Below are two ways of making rehydration drink. If you can, add half a cup of fruit juice, coconut water, or mashed ripe banana to either drink. These contain potassium, a mineral which helps a sick person accept more food and drink.

Give the child sips of this drink every 5 minutes, day and night, until he begins to urinate normally. A large person needs 3 or more liters a day. A small child usually needs at least 1 liter a day, or 1 glass for each watery stool. Keep giving the drink often, and in small sips. Even if the person vomits, not all of the drink will be vomited.

Made with powdered cereal and salt.
(Powdered rice is best. But you can use finely ground maize, wheat flour, sorghum, or cooked and mashed potatoes.)

In 1 liter of clean WATER put half of a level teaspoon of SALT,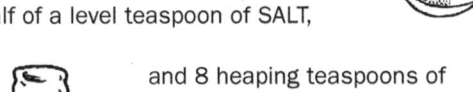

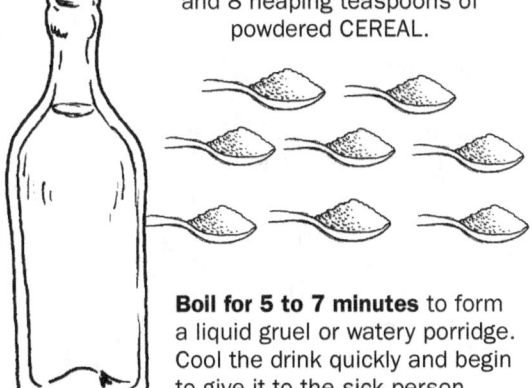

and 8 heaping teaspoons of powdered CEREAL.

Boil for 5 to 7 minutes to form a liquid gruel or watery porridge. Cool the drink quickly and begin to give it to the sick person.

CAUTION: Taste the drink each time before you give it to make sure that it has not spoiled. Cereal drinks can spoil within a few hours in hot weather.

Made with sugar and salt.
(You can use raw, brown sugar or molasses instead of white sugar.)

In 1 liter of clean WATER put half of a level teaspoon of SALT,

and 8 level teaspoons of SUGAR. Mix well.

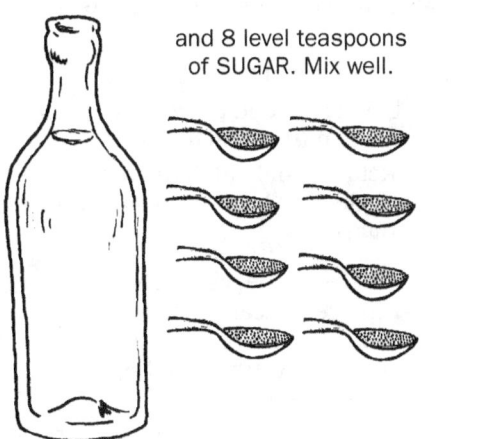

CAUTION: Before adding the sugar, taste the drink and be sure it is less salty than tears.

WARNING: If dehydration gets worse or other danger signs appear, get medical help.

Hand-washing with soap and water

One of the best ways to prevent diarrhea diseases is to wash hands **after** defecating or handling babies' feces, and **before** preparing food, feeding children, or eating.

Keeping a source of clean water near your home will make hand-washing much easier. But washing with water alone is not enough. To make hand-washing effective, use soap to remove dirt and germs. If no soap is available, use sand, soil, or ashes.

Rub hands together well with soap and flowing water like that from a pump, faucet, or tippy-tap.

Count to 30 as you scrub your hands all over. Then rub hands together under the water to rinse off soap, sand, or ashes. Dry with a clean cloth or let your hands dry in the air.

The tippy-tap: A simple hand-washing device

The tippy-tap is a simple device that allows people to wash hands with very little water. It also allows the user to rub his or her hands together while water runs over them. It is made of materials that are available at no cost in most places and can be put wherever people need to wash their hands: near the cooking stove, at the toilet, or in rural food stores, for example.

How to make a plastic tippy-tap

To make this tippy-tap you need 1) a plastic bottle with a screw-on cap, of the sort that soda drinks come in, and 2) the inside tube from a ball-point pen, or some other small, stiff, hollow tube.

1.   Clean the bottle.
2.   Using a heated piece of wire, make a small hole in the lower part of the bottle.
3.   Remove and clean the inside tube from a ball-point pen. Cut it off at an angle, and push it through the hole in the bottle. The tube should fit tightly.

4.   Fill the bottle with water and replace the cap. When the cap is tight, no water should flow through the tube. When the cap is loose, water should flow out in a steady stream. When you are sure that it works, hang it or place it on a shelf where people can use it for hand-washing. Keep soap nearby, or thread a bar of soap with string and tie it to the bottle.

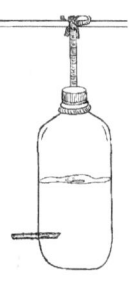

5.   To use the tippy-tap: Loosen the cap just enough to let water flow. Wet your hands, add soap, and rub your hands together under the water until they are clean.

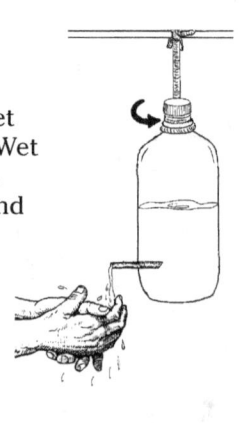

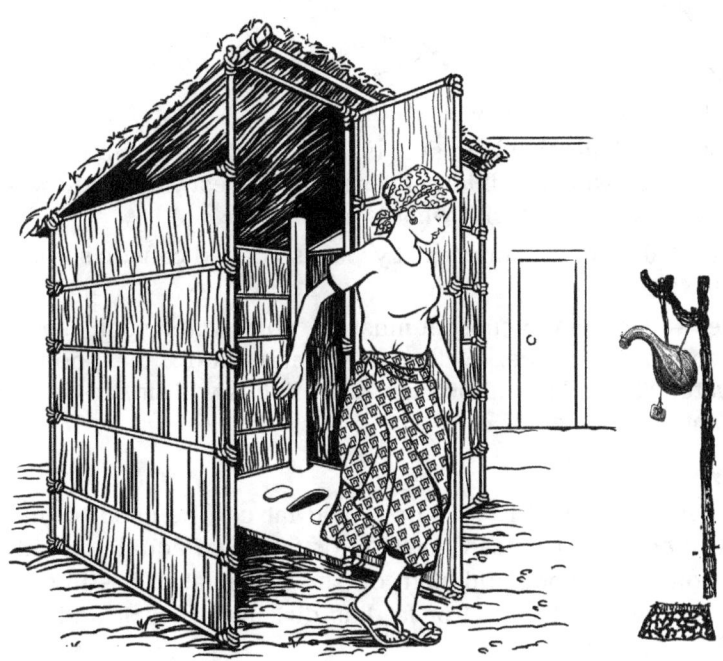

Tippy-taps can also be made with different designs
and from different materials. Another that is
common is made from a dried calabash gourd.

Sanitary use of water for toilet hygiene

In many places people wash their bottoms with water after defecating. This anal washing is a very effective way to stay clean. But because the water used gets contaminated with feces, it must be disposed of carefully. Never dispose of it into a stream or lake. Empty the container into a toilet or into a waste pit at least 20 meters from any surface water, wells, or springs. The container must be kept clean too.

- Refill the container with wash water often. Do not let it go unwashed for more than a day. The longer it sits, the more germs grow in and on it.
- Wash the container with soap or ashes every time before you fill it.
- The container used for anal washing should be stored away from other water containers and away from places where food is prepared.
- Wash your hands well after the last time you touch the container — germs are sure to be on its handle and surfaces!

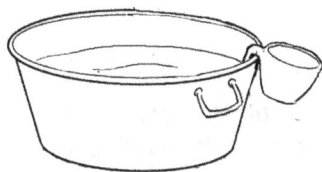

How to make soap

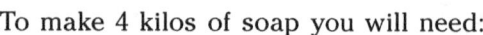

Basic ingredients

To make 4 kilos of soap you will need:

- Oil or fat — 3 liters (13 cups) of oil or 2.75 kilos (6 pounds) of hard fat. Different oils and fats will give different results. The best way to know what fat or oil to use is to experiment with what is available.
- Lye — 370 grams (13 ounces). Lye is also called caustic soda or sodium hydroxide.
- Water — 1.2 liters (5 cups). It must be "soft" water, such as rain or spring water. To "soften" hard water (well or river water), add ¼ teaspoon of lye for each liter of water. Stir and let sit for a few days. Solids will sink to the bottom. Pour off the softened water for use.

Using dirty or rancid fat

Fresh oil or fat is costly. Dirty oil or rancid fat can be used to make soap, but must be cleaned first. To clean, melt oil or fat in an equal amount of water and bring to a boil. Let it cool, and skim off the oil or fat. If it still smells bad, do it again with new water. If the oil or fat has dirt in it, melt it and pour it through a fine cloth until it is clean.

Perfume

Perfume or essential oils give soap an attractive scent. For 4 kilos of soap, use one of the following: 4 teaspoons of sassafras oil, 2 teaspoons of citronella or lavender oil, or 1 teaspoon of clove or lemon oil. For soap that promotes healthy skin, add 1 or 2 teaspoons of oil of neem, moringa, jatropha, or baobab.

Equipment

- 2 large pots, bowls, or buckets made of stainless steel, fired clay, or cast iron. Do not use equipment made from aluminum because the lye will damage it.
- A bowl or other clean container big enough to hold all the fat.
- Wooden spoons or stirring sticks.
- Measuring cups.

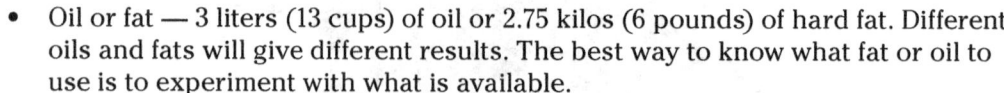

- An accurate weighing scale (lye is measured by weight).
- Molds: the best molds are shallow wooden boxes that have no openings on the bottom or sides but are open on the top, and can be pulled apart gently. Molds can also be made from small gourds or coconut shells.
  - Use cloth or waxed paper to line the molds so that soap can be easily removed.

> **WARNING:** **Lye can burn the skin and eyes.** To be safe, it must combine with the fat and set for several weeks. While making soap, wear safety glasses, long gloves, clothes that cover the arms and legs, and closed shoes. If you get burned by lye, wash the skin right away with cold water, then put on citrus juice or vinegar to cool and disinfect the burn.

Recipe

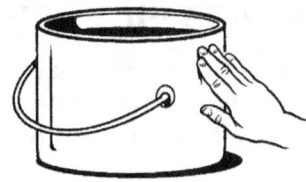

1. Add lye to water – never the other way around. The mixture will heat up. Let it cool to body temperature. Do not put fingers in the solution or it will burn. To test the temperature, feel the outside of the container.

2. Melt any solid fat in the oil/fat mixture.

3. Pour the lye water slowly into the oil/fat mixture, stirring it constantly in one direction. Then add perfume or essential oil. The mixture must be stirred for at least half an hour after all the lye has been added. The mixture should become thicker. When the spoon causes lines to appear on top of the thick solution, it is ready to pour in the molds.

4. Pour the mixture into lined molds and leave to set undisturbed for 2 days. If it has not set or if it has grease on top, leave it longer.

5. When the soap has set, remove it from the molds and cut it into bars using a knife or a wire.

6. Stack the bars on trays and let them sit for 4 to 6 weeks. Do not use the soap too soon – it still burns!

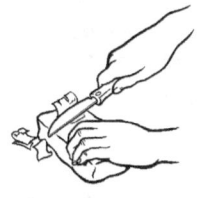

7. When the soap is finished, you can shave it from the bar in curls. Touch the soap to the tip of your tongue to check its quality. If it has a slight bite or burn, it is good. Cover the soap so it does not lose moisture.

Problems?

If it is very sharp and burns, there is too much lye. If it has no bite, there is not enough lye. If the soap you made was not successful, it may have been because:

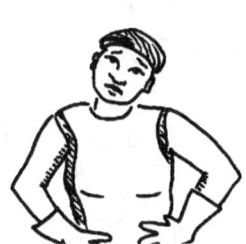

*   The fat or oil was rancid or dirty and not cleaned enough.
*   The lye water was too hot or too cold when it was poured into the oil/fat mixture.
*   The mixture was stirred too fast or not long enough.

If the soap is not good, try again:

*   Cut the soap into bits. Put it in a pot with 12 cups (2.8 liters) of water. Use gloves to touch the soap.
*   Bring it slowly to a boil. Boil for 10 minutes, stirring at times.
*   If the soap had too little lye (no bite at all), add a small amount of lye. If the soap had too much lye (sharp bite), add some pre-boiled, strained and cooled fat. Stir until the spoon causes lines to appear on top of the thick solution.
*   Pour into molds. Let stand 48 hours. Cut into bars, stack the bars on trays and let them sit for 4 to 6 weeks.

Community education activity: Preventing diarrhea

The next 2 pages have a drawing activity to learn about how diarrhea diseases spread and how to prevent them from spreading. After doing these activities, it may be useful to read and discuss pages 6, 7, and 8.

HOW DIARRHEA DISEASES SPREAD

This activity helps to explain how germs that cause diarrhea pass from person to person. People make drawings and put them together to form a 'story' about how diarrhea spreads.

Time: 1 to 1 ½ hours

Materials: small drawing paper, large drawing paper, colored pens or markers, sticky tape, sample drawings.

➡ **Step 1:** Form groups of 5 to 8 people. Each person draws a picture that shows something about how she thinks people get diarrhea. Each drawing should show just one part of the story of how diarrhea spreads. If a person has difficulty drawing, she can write a word instead or get help from someone else. It may help to have sample drawings to stimulate the group discussion.

➡ **Step 2:** Within each group, each person shows her or his drawing. The other people in the group tell what they see. This is to make sure that every person understands the drawings.

➡ **Step 3:** Each group puts their drawings in an order that makes a story about how germs spread. If the group sees that there are drawings missing, they can make new drawings to fit the story. When the drawings are in order, they are taped to a larger piece of paper. Arrows can be drawn between the drawings to make a chart that tells the story of how germs spread.

➡ **Step 4:** Each group shows its chart to the other groups. The group showing the drawings tells the 'story' of how diarrhea passes from one person to another.

➡ **Step 5:** The whole group now has a discussion about the activity. Is every group's story the same? How are the stories different? Why? Talk about the ways diarrhea can spread. How do economic and social conditions put people at risk? What behaviors and beliefs put people at risk of infection? What other ways do diseases spread that were not illustrated in the activity?

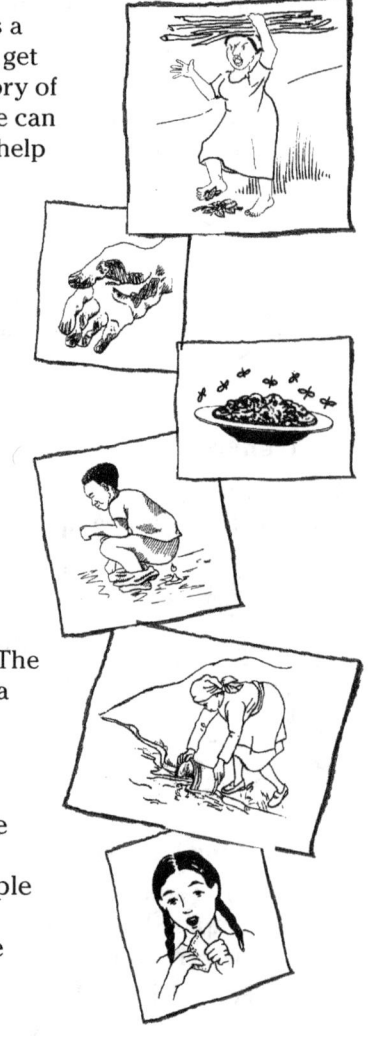

This activity can be used to talk about other health problems as well, like parasites, cholera, malaria, and HIV/AIDS.

BLOCKING THE SPREAD OF DIARRHEA

This activity uses the stories from the last activity to show how to prevent or 'block' diarrhea from being spread.

Time: 30 minutes to 1 hour

Materials: large sheet of drawing paper, colored pens or markers, sticky tape, story charts from the activity called "How Diarrhea Diseases Spread."

➡ **Step 1:** Work in the same small groups as in the activity called "How Diarrhea Diseases Spread." Each group looks at the pictures from "How Diarrhea Diseases Spread." They then talk about how to stop the spread of disease by washing hands, using toilets, protecting food and water, and so on. Each of these actions is a 'barrier' that blocks the spread of diarrhea.

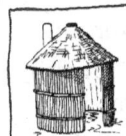

➡ **Step 2:** When the group has agreed on what barriers will stop the spread of germs, each person draws a picture that shows one way to stop the spread of diarrhea diseases.

➡ **Step 3:** The group then talks about how to change the story from "How diarrhea diseases spread" to "How to stop diarrhea." Where do the new drawings fit in the story so that they will stop the spread of illness? The new drawings are taped in place in the old story to show how the story can change.

➡ **Step 4:** Each group shows its new stories. The whole group talks about which disease barriers they use and which ones they do not use. Do all the disease barriers work all the time? Why, or why not? Why is it hard to use some of these barriers? How can the community work together to make sure that diarrhea diseases do not spread?

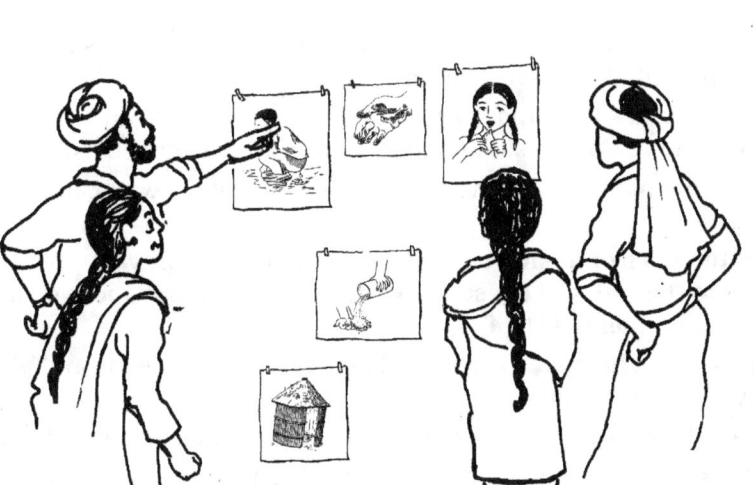

Planning for sanitation

Every person and every community has a way of dealing with sanitation, even if it just means that people go into the bush or forest to urinate and defecate. Households and communities can benefit from talking about the sanitation methods that will work best for everyone.

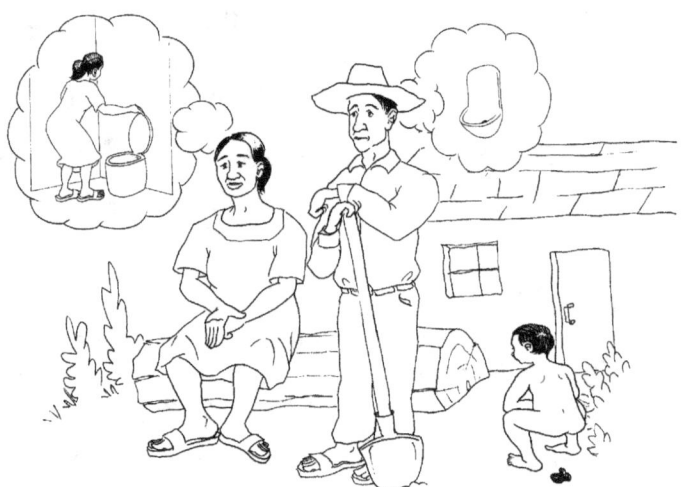

A sanitation plan that leaves women or anyone else without toilets will not prevent illness in the community.

Healthy sanitation must consider the needs of children, who cannot take care of themselves. It must also ensure that women have toilets that they feel safe using and a way to keep clean during monthly bleeding.

Small steps to sustainable sanitation

In any community — and even in a single household — there may be several sanitation methods in use at one time. Some people may want to change the way they take care of their sanitation needs, while others may not. Whether it means building a new kind of toilet, helping to meet the needs of those without access to safe toilets, or some other kind of change, almost every sanitation method can be improved.

Small, step-by-step changes are easier than big changes all at once. Examples of small changes that can have a big impact on health, safety, and comfort are:

- keeping wash water and soap near the toilet
- adding a vent to a pit toilet
- adding a durable platform to an open pit

When planning or making changes in the way human waste is disposed of in your community, keep in mind that every method should:

- **Prevent disease** – it should keep disease-carrying waste and insects away from people, both at the site of the toilet and in nearby homes.
- **Protect water supplies** – it should not pollute drinking water, surface water, or *groundwater.*
- **Protect the environment** – ecological sanitation can prevent pollution, return *nutrients* to the soil, and conserve water. (To learn more about ecological sanitation, see pages 33 to 43.)
- **Be simple and affordable** – it should fit local people's needs and abilities, and be easy to clean and maintain.
- **Be culturally acceptable** – it should fit local customs, beliefs, and desires.
- **Work for everyone** – it should address the health needs of children and adults, of women and men.

Sanitation decisions are community decisions

When decisions about toilets are made by the people who will use them, it is more likely that people's different sanitation needs will be met. And because household, neighborhood, and village sanitation decisions can affect people downstream, when neighboring communities work together, health can improve for everyone.

Community participation can make the difference between success and failure when a government or outside agency tries to improve sanitation. When local people participate in sanitation planning, the result is more likely to fit local needs.

In 1992, the government of El Salvador spent over US$10 million to build thousands of toilets. These toilets were meant to turn waste into fertilizer, but they needed more care and cleaning than the old toilets local people were used to. The government did not involve anyone in the communities to help build them and there was no training in how to use them, so people did not learn how they worked.

After the project was finished, the government studied how the toilets were being used. They learned that many of the toilets were not being used well, and others were not used at all.

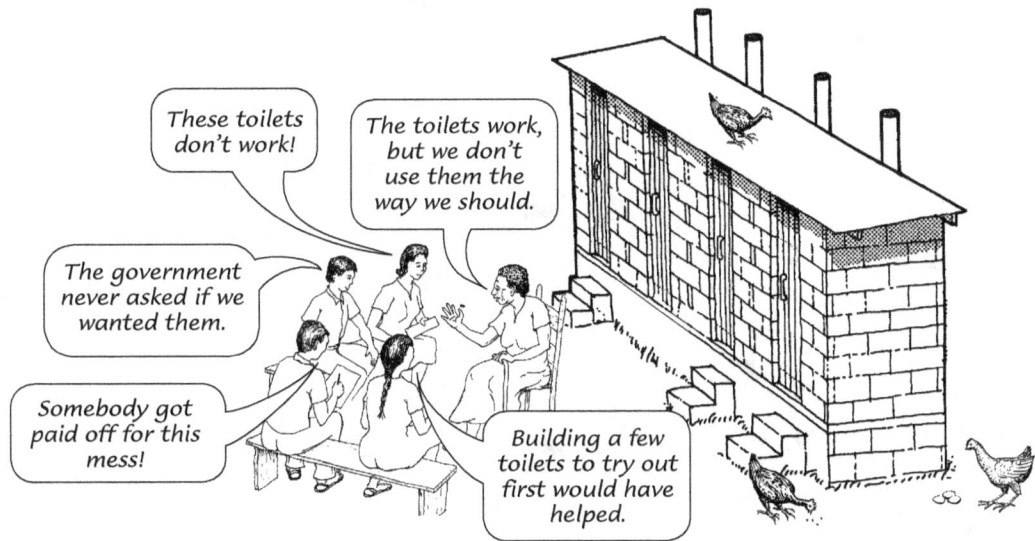

When people participate in planning, the result is more likely to fit their needs.

Someone must clean the toilet

No one likes to clean the toilet. But someone has to do it.

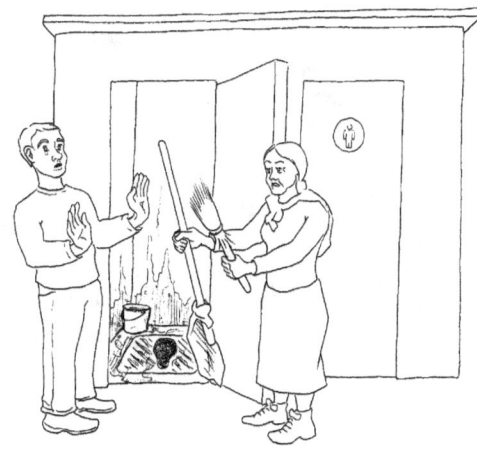

Often, the job of planning, building, and fixing toilets is considered men's work or work for specialists. But the less pleasant and more constant task of cleaning toilets often falls to women or people of lower social classes. It is unfair if tasks that are necessary but unpleasant always fall to people with no voice in making decisions. And in the long run, it can lead to these tasks being done poorly, or not being done at all.

Sharing unpleasant tasks is a way to ensure that the work gets done, though it often creates social conflicts.

Contamination upstream causes illness downstream

It is easy to talk about participation and cooperation in the household or community, but it can be very hard to do. And it is difficult when people who did not create a problem must fix it.

Drawing for discussion: What threats to good health do you see?

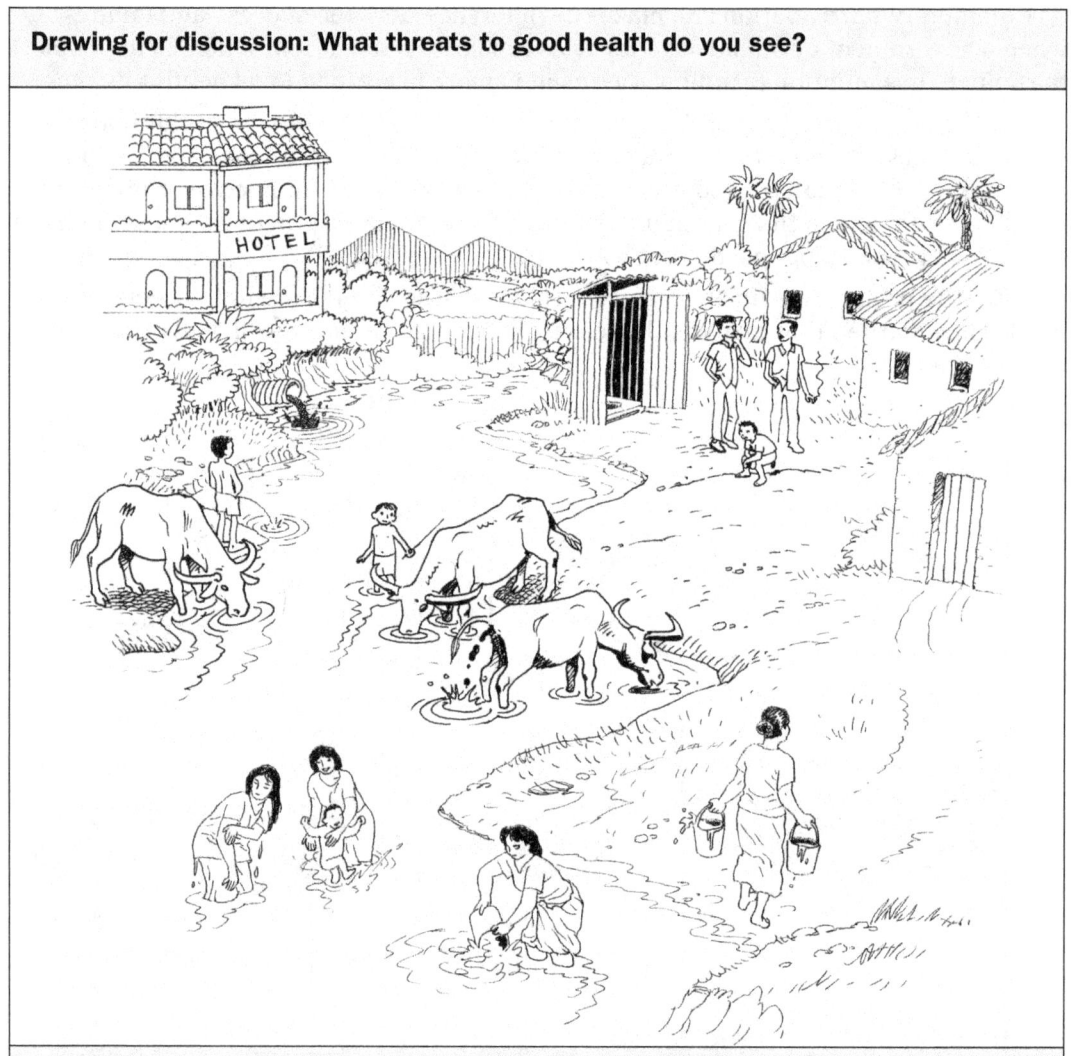

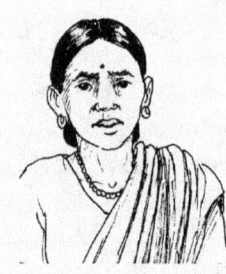

Health worker discussion questions:

- What kinds of water use are shown here?
- How do people's sanitation activities affect the water they use?
- How is people's health affected by these activities?
- What could people in the picture do to protect their health?
- How can these people work together to improve sanitation for all?

Women and men have different sanitation needs

Women and men have different needs and customs when it comes to using the toilet. Men may be more comfortable than women relieving themselves in public or open spaces. Women have a greater share of family work such as caring for children, collecting water and firewood, cooking, and cleaning. All of these things affect their access to toilets that are safe, clean, comfortable, and private.

Addressing women's needs often challenges traditional ideas about how decisions are made. Because it may be difficult to make or accept changes, it takes time and effort by both men and women to improve health for everyone. The activity on page 22 can help promote discussion about some of the problems women have gaining access to safe sanitation.

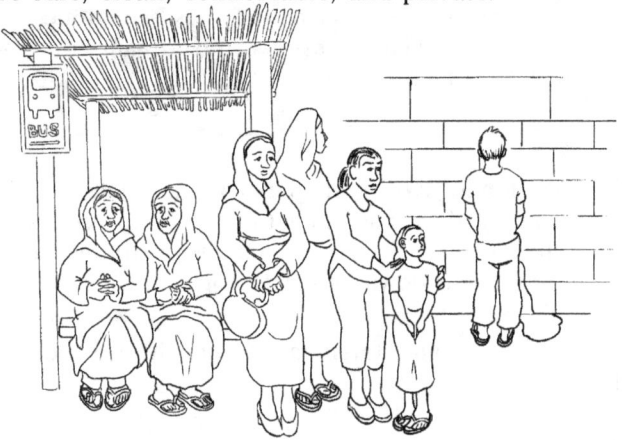

It is generally easier for men to relieve themselves than it is for women.

Planning toilets with women's needs in mind

Leaving women out of sanitation planning puts them at a greater risk of health problems because it is less likely that their needs will be met. When women do not have the money, resources, power, or confidence to ensure that their needs are met, this increases their burden even more.

Men must keep women's needs in mind and provide incentives for women to participate in community sanitation planning in a way that does not simply give them more work to do:

- Organize meetings at times when women can participate.
- Ensure that women are invited to speak out and can feel comfortable speaking out.
- Have separate meetings for women if that makes it easier for women to speak up.
- Share decision-making power.

Women usually teach and care for children. When women's needs are not met, the needs of children may be unmet as well. When women are not included in planning household and community sanitation, the whole community suffers.

> *If you teach a man, you teach one person. If you teach a woman, you teach a whole nation.*
> *— African proverb*

REMOVING THE BARRIER TO TOILETS FOR WOMEN

This activity helps people talk about issues that may prevent women from having access to safe and healthy toilets. The goal is to decide what changes might be necessary to improve health for everyone. After the activity has been done with just women, a session can be organized with both men and women.

 Time: 1 to 1 ½ hours

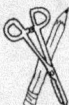 **Materials:** flip chart or large drawing paper, pens, sticky tape.

➡ **Step 1.** Write statements about toilets on a flipchart or large piece of paper. Then read each statement to the group, and ask each person to decide whether she agrees or disagrees. (Ask people to raise a hand if they agree, or to leave their hands down if they do not.) For every 'yes' answer, make a mark next to the phrase.

Here are some statements that might be used.

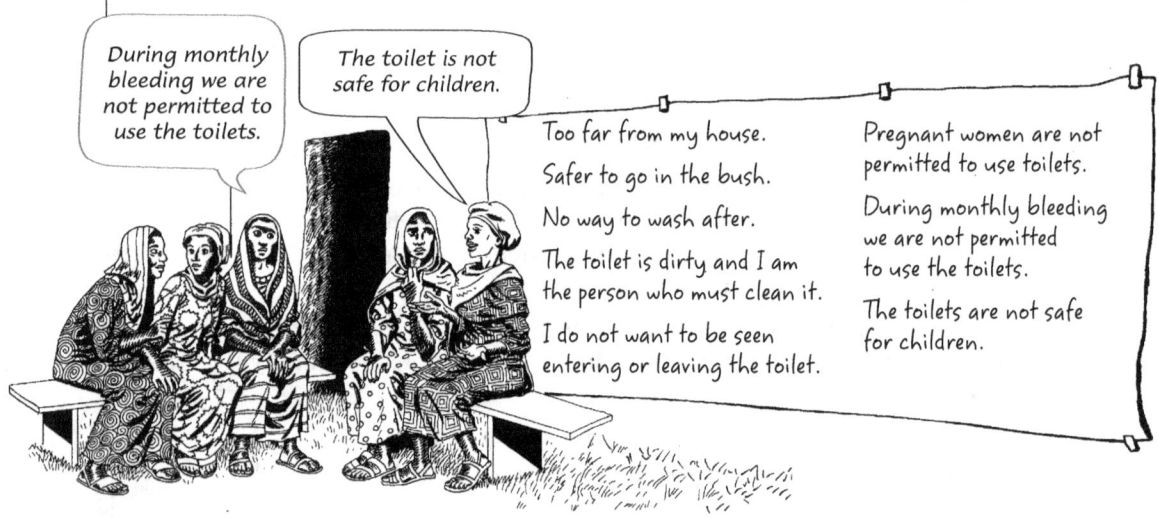

During monthly bleeding we are not permitted to use the toilets.

The toilet is not safe for children.

Too far from my house.

Safer to go in the bush.

No way to wash after.

The toilet is dirty and I am the person who must clean it.

I do not want to be seen entering or leaving the toilet.

Pregnant women are not permitted to use toilets.

During monthly bleeding we are not permitted to use the toilets.

The toilets are not safe for children.

➡ **Step 2.** Count the marks beside each statement. Choose the problems that were mentioned most often and begin a discussion about them. What is the cause of the problem? What illnesses may result from this problem? What can be done to improve the situation? What are the barriers to improving the situation?

➡ **Step 3.** End with the group deciding on some actions that can be taken by both men and women to ensure that everyone's needs are met.

Making toilets easier to use

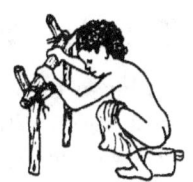

There are many ways to make toilets easier for children and adults with disabilities to use. People need different adaptations depending on their abilities, so it is best to involve people with disabilities in planning. Be creative in finding solutions that meet everyone's needs.

If a person has **difficulty squatting**, make a simple hand support or a raised seat. Or if the toilet is set in the ground, make a hole in the seat or a chair or stool and place it over the toilet.

If a person has **difficulty controlling her body**, make supports for her back, sides, and legs, and a seat belt or bar.

removable front bar can be added if needed →

Use a rope or fence to guide **blind** people from the house to the toilet.

If a person has **difficulty adjusting clothing**, adapt the clothing to make it loose or elastic. Make a clean, dry place to lie down and dress.

If a person has **difficulty sitting** you can make moveable handrails and steps.

Adapt a toilet for wheelchair users

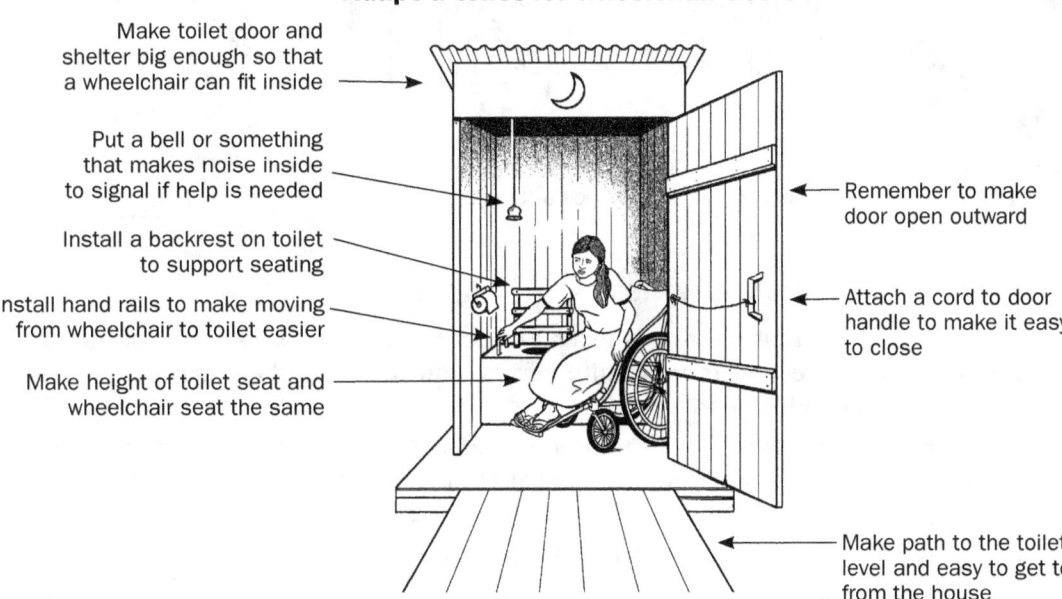

Make toilet door and shelter big enough so that a wheelchair can fit inside →

Put a bell or something that makes noise inside to signal if help is needed

Install a backrest on toilet to support seating

Install hand rails to make moving from wheelchair to toilet easier

Make height of toilet seat and wheelchair seat the same

← Remember to make door open outward

← Attach a cord to door handle to make it easy to close

← Make path to the toilet level and easy to get to from the house

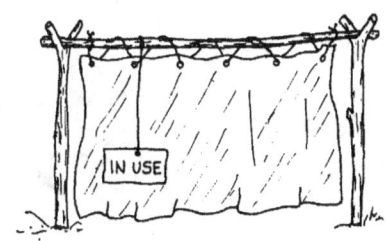

IN USE

Remember, a person with a disability feels the same need for privacy as anyone else and should get the privacy he or she needs.

Toilets for children's health

Children have a high risk of illness from poor
sanitation. While adults may live with diarrhea diseases
and worms, children die from these illnesses.

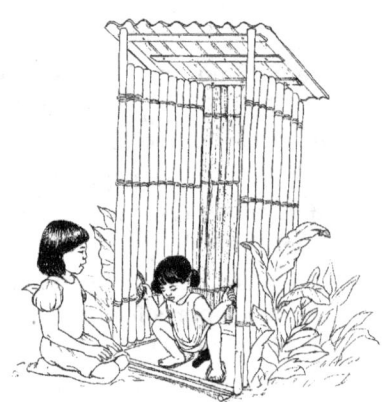

When children have toilets they feel safe using and
have an easy way to stay clean, they get sick less. Pit
toilets can be dangerous and frightening for small
children because of the darkness and the large hole.
Many children, especially girls, leave school because
schools lack safe toilets.

Allowing children to help build toilets and teaching
them about illness caused by poor sanitation are some
ways to help them develop healthy behaviors.

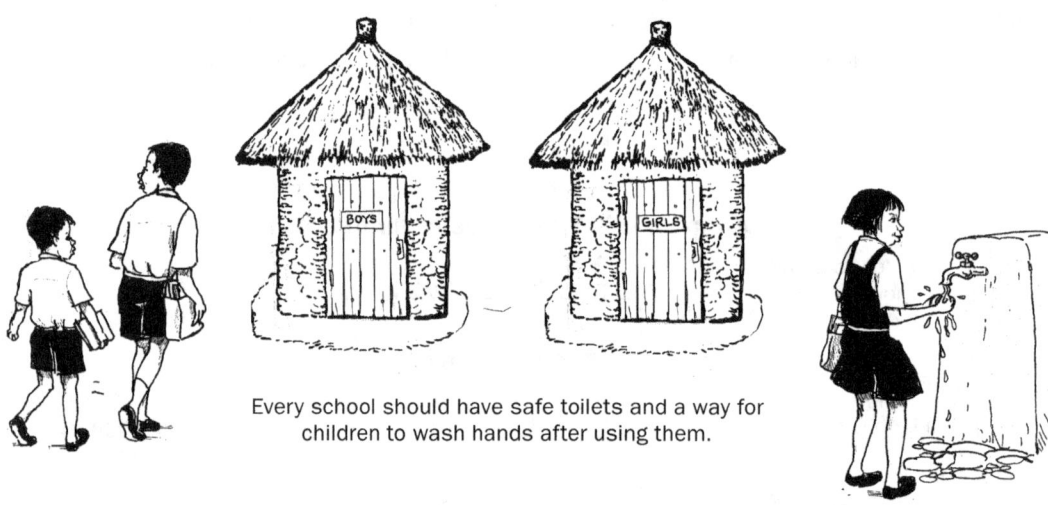

Every school should have safe toilets and a way for
children to wash hands after using them.

Helping small children stay clean

Many people believe that children's feces are not as dangerous as those of adults.
This is not true. All feces carry harmful germs, and handling them can cause
serious illness in children and adults.

In rural areas, parents can help children too small to use a toilet by making a hole
near the house, and adding a handful of soil after each use. It is also important to:

- Wash babies and young children after they defecate.
- Wash your hands after handling babies' feces.
- Bury the feces or put them in a safe toilet.
- Wash soiled clothes away from drinking water sources.

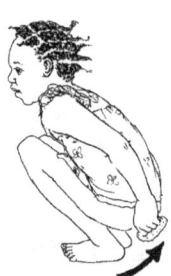

Teach boys and girls to wipe or wash carefully and to wash
their hands after using the toilet. Girls especially should be
taught to wipe from front to back. Wiping forward can spread
germs into the urinary opening and the vagina, causing
bladder infections and other health problems.

Sanitation for cities and towns

In cities and towns that lack sufficient water and toilets, health problems can spread very quickly. It is difficult to improve sanitation services in crowded cities and towns without a lot of help from governments, NGOs, and other development partners. This book can only offer some guidelines to help think about possible solutions.

The main barriers to good sanitation services in cities are:

- **Physical.** Often, sanitation is considered only after neighborhoods and settlements have roads, electricity, and water. Once a city is built, it is much harder to plan for and build sanitation services.
- **Economic.** Sewer systems and public toilets are costly to build and maintain. If there is little government support, it is difficult to afford sanitation.
- **Political.** Local governments may not want to deliver services to informal settlements and poorer neighborhoods. And there may be laws that prevent people from planning and building their own toilets and sewage systems.
- **Cultural.** People and officials in cities often want flush toilets and costly sewer systems, making it difficult to agree on more sustainable and affordable alternatives.

Planning for urban sanitation is made easier when:

- people have choices that fit their different needs.
- community groups take the lead in developing solutions that are appropriate and affordable.
- people's human right to have water is recognized.
- the needs of the most vulnerable groups are taken into account.
- partnerships are built among communities, non-governmental organizations, local governments, and businesses. For these partnerships to work well, they must be controlled by those most in need of sanitation improvements – the communities themselves.

Sanitation for emergencies

In emergency settlements such as refugee camps, sanitation is a first priority. Simple defecation trenches and pit toilets can be made quickly using local materials. One trench or pit toilet for each family, or for a small group of families, will allow for the most comfortable use.

Sanitation trenches and pit toilets should be built downhill and away from water sources, but close enough to family settlements that people do not have to walk long distances to use them.

This shallow trench latrine is easier to dig than a pit toilet or a deep trench. It has shelves for the feet to make it easier to use than a simple trench. The trench is about 30 centimeters deep. Each user covers his or her feces with a small amount of soil. A portable shelter can be built to give privacy and to protect users from rain. Special care should be taken to assure women's privacy and safety.

When it is full, cover the trench completely with soil. Plants and trees will benefit from the rich soil.

Urban community sanitation

Not long ago, Yoff was a typical West African fishing village outside of Dakar, the capital city of Senegal. Families lived in compounds connected by walking paths and open spaces. But as Dakar grew and swallowed Yoff, it became part of a large urban area with an international airport and a lot of car traffic.

As the town grew, many houses installed flush toilets connected to open pits where the sewage sat and bred disease. Other people, too poor to afford toilets, used open sandy areas to fulfill their needs. But with many people living close together, this quickly became a health problem.

A town development committee came together to solve the sanitation problem. They began by looking at the resources they had: strong community networks, skilled builders, and people committed to keeping village life. They also had some new ideas about ecological sanitation.

In the village, houses were grouped around open common areas where people could gather and talk. After talking to many villagers, the committee made a plan to use this open area for a sanitation system that would make the area more attractive, rather than uglier. Instead of promoting household toilets and underground sewage tanks, they would promote community ecological sanitation.

The committee worked with residents to build urine-diverting dry toilets. Each set of toilets would be shared by the whole compound. The urine would run through pipes into beds of reeds. The feces, after being dried out, would be used to fertilize trees. All of this would help to keep the village green. Local masons and builders were hired to construct the toilets and to maintain the common areas.

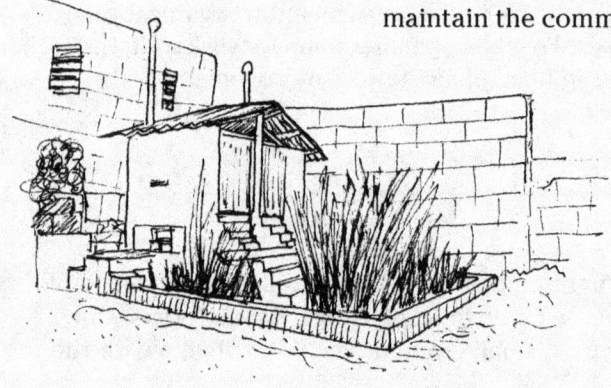

This urban sanitation project not only prevented health problems – it helped to preserve the way the people of Yoff wanted to live.

Creative solutions for healthier cities

Urban sanitation does not have to use large, expensive, water-based sewage systems. Water-based sanitation systems produce large amounts of dirty water that must be treated before it can be reused. If it is not purified – and it usually is not – it can lead to contamination of drinking and bathing water, contamination of land used for housing and farming, and other serious environmental and health problems.

If urban sanitation services are combined with urban farming, parks, garbage collection, and energy production, cities can become healthier and more beautiful places to live. When community groups work with local governments to come up with creative solutions, the result will be greener, healthier cities.

Toilet choices

In the rest of this booklet, we describe several kinds of toilets that can be built using local resources. No one toilet design is right for every community or household, so it is important to understand the benefits of each choice.

Note: These drawings show toilets with no doors and covers so you can see inside them, but all toilets need doors and covers.

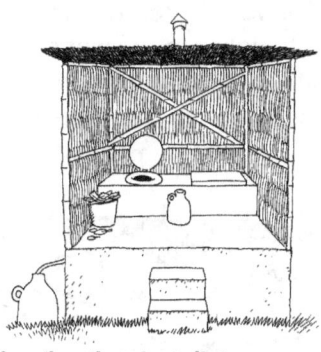

Urine-diverting dry toilet

An above-ground structure with two chambers, a toilet bowl that separates urine and feces, and a pipe that diverts urine. Best in places where people will use treated human waste as fertilizer, and where the groundwater is high or there is risk of flooding. (See page 37.)

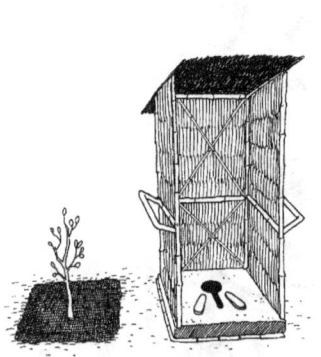

Simple compost toilet for tree planting

A shallow pit, a platform, and a movable shelter.Best in places where people wish to plant trees and can manage a movable toilet. (See page 35.)

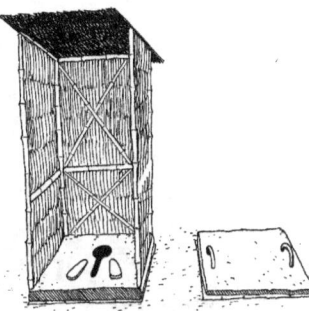

2-pit compost toilet

2 shallow pits, a platform, and a light, movable shelter or a permanent shelter big enough for both pits. Best in places where people will use treated human waste as fertilizer. (See page 36.)

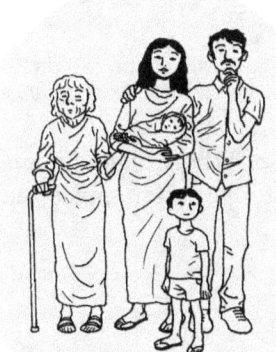

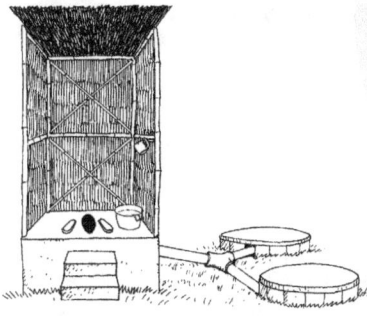

Pour-flush toilet

A water-seal trap, a platform, 1 or 2 deep pits, and a shelter. Best in places with deep groundwater and where people use water for anal washing after using the toilet. (See page 44.)

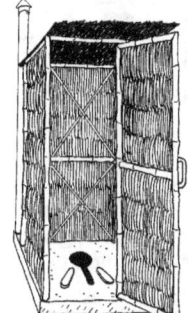

Ventilated improved pit toilet

A deep pit, a concrete or wood and earth platform, a shelter, and a vent pipe to trap flies. Best in places with deep groundwater and no risk of flooding. (See page 32.)

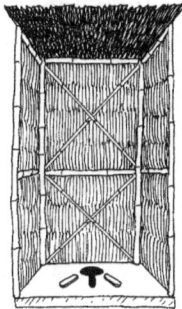

Closed pit toilet

A deep pit, a platform, and a shelter. Best in places with deep groundwater and no risk of flooding. (See page 29.)

Where to build a toilet

When deciding where to build a toilet, make sure you will not pollute wells or groundwater. The risk of groundwater pollution depends on local conditions such as the type of soil, the amount of moisture in the area, and the depth of the groundwater. But some general rules can help ensure safety.

The bottom of the pit (if it is a pit toilet) or the chamber (if it is a compost toilet) should be at least 2 ½ meters above the groundwater. If you dig a pit for a toilet and the soil is very wet, or if the pit fills with water, this is a bad place to put a toilet. Keep in mind that water levels are much higher in the wet season than in the dry season. Do not build pit toilets on ground that gets flooded.

When there is a risk of groundwater pollution from pit toilets, consider building an above-ground toilet, such as the dry toilet on page 37.

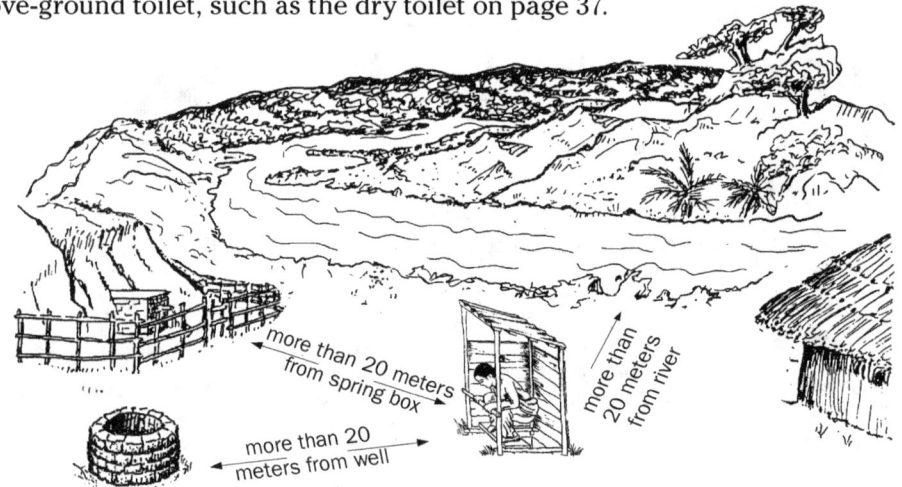

A toilet should be at least 20 meters from water
sources (rivers, lakes, springs, streams and wells).

Groundwater flows downhill. So, if there is no choice but to build a toilet in a place where there is a risk of groundwater pollution, place the toilet downhill from nearby wells.

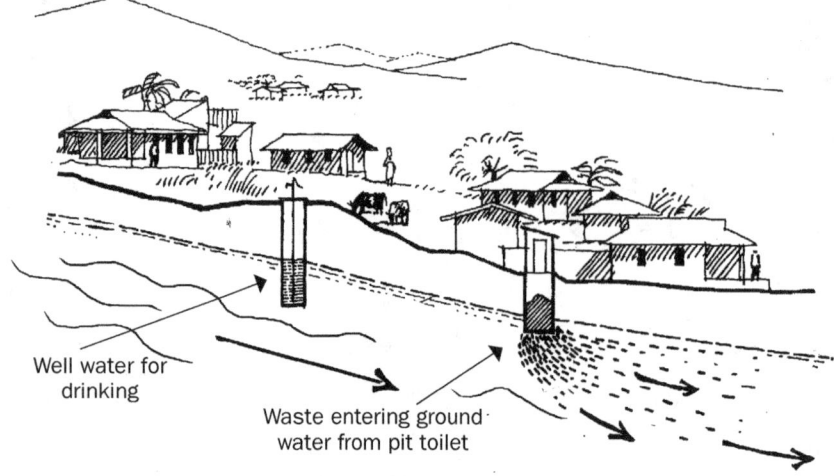

Wells should be uphill from pit toilets because
groundwater flows downhill.

Closed pit toilets

A closed pit toilet has a platform with a hole in it and a lid to cover the hole when it is not in use. The platform can be made of wood, concrete, or logs covered with earth. Concrete platforms keep water out and last many years. A closed pit toilet should also have a lining or concrete ring beam to prevent the platform or the pit itself from collapsing. (To make a concrete platform and ring beam, see pages 30 and 31.)

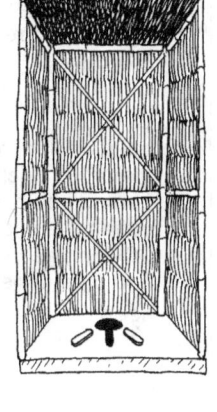

The ventilated improved pit toilet shown on page 32 uses a vent pipe to reduce smells and flies.

A problem with pit toilets is that once the pit is full, the toilet can no longer be used. One way to take advantage of the waste in full pits is to plant a tree on the site. To do this, remove the platform, ring beam, and shelter, and cover the waste with 30 centimeters (2 hands-widths) of soil mixed with dry plant matter. Allow several months for the waste to settle, fill it with more soil, and plant a tree.

Another option is to add soil frequently while in use and let it sit for 2 years to allow the waste to *decompose*. Then dig it out, use the waste as fertilizer, and use the pit again. Always wash hands after handling and digging the soil around toilets

To make a closed pit toilet

1. Dig a hole less than 1 meter across and at least 2 meters deep.

2. Line the top of the pit with stones, brick, concrete or other material that will support a platform and prevent the pit from collapsing. A concrete ring beam works well (see page 31).

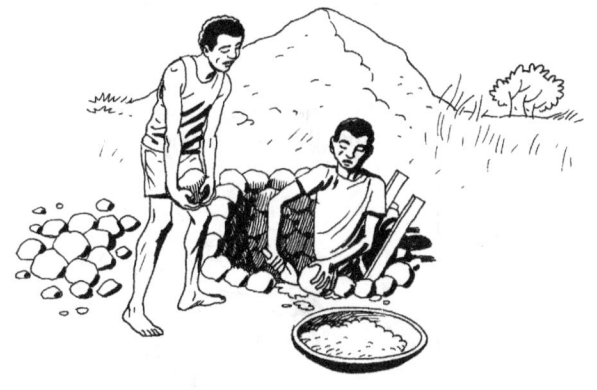

3. Make a platform and a shelter to put over the pit. A concrete platform works best, but local materials like logs or bamboo and mud can work too. If you make a platform from logs, use wood that does not rot easily.

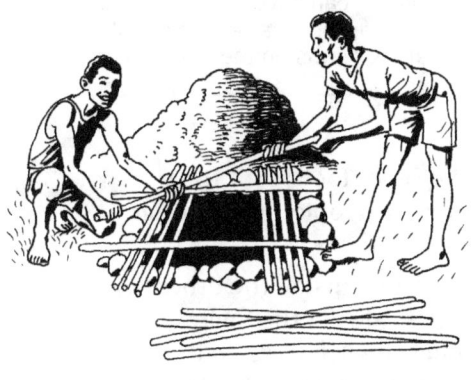

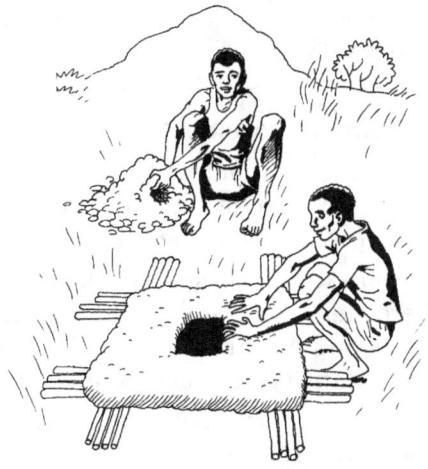

How to make a concrete toilet platform

A well-made concrete platform will last many years. One 50 kilo bag of cement is enough to make 4 platforms or 2 platforms and 2 ring beams (see page 31). You will also need reinforcing wires, bricks, and boards to form the mold, and a piece of wood cut to the shape of a keyhole to mold the hole. This platform is square, but you could make a round one.

1. Lay down a plastic sheet or used cement bags on flat ground. On top of this, make a mold of bricks or boards about 120 centimeters long, 90 centimeters wide and 6 centimeters deep.

2. Place a wooden "keyhole" mold in the center, to shape the toilet hole. You can also use bricks to block out the hole, and shape the hole after the concrete is poured.

3. Make a concrete mix of 1 part cement, 2 parts gravel, 3 parts sand, and enough water so it is wet but holds together. Pour the concrete into the mold until it is half-way to the top.

4. Place reinforcing wires 3 millimeters thick on top of the wet concrete. Use 4 to 6 wires going in each direction. Make handles of wire 8 to 10 millimeters thick, and set them in the concrete near the corners.

5. Pour the rest of the concrete, and smooth it with a block of wood.

6. Remove the keyhole mold when the concrete begins to harden (after about 3 hours). If you used a brick mold, remove the bricks and form the hole into a keyhole shape. Leave the slab overnight and cover it with wet cement sacks, damp cloth or a plastic sheet. Wet it several times a day to keep it damp for 7 days. Keeping it wet lets the concrete harden slowly and become strong.

7. When the concrete is hardened, place the platform over the pit. To make the pit more secure, also use a concrete ring beam (see page 31).

8. Make a cover for the hole out of concrete or wood. It can have a handle, or can be made to be moved by a person's foot, to avoid getting germs on the hands.

Platform improvements

Because germs and worms can collect near the hole, foot rests to stand on will reduce the risk of health problems. If people prefer to sit, make a round hole and a concrete seat.

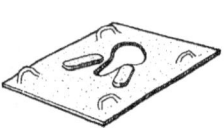

To make a mold, use 2 buckets of different sizes, one inside the other. There must be several inches of space between the sides of the inner bucket and the outer bucket. Weight the inner bucket with rocks so it stays on the bottom, and pour concrete into the space between buckets.

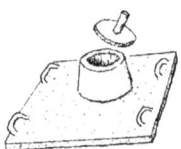

To make a dry toilet, you can use this platform with a urine-separating toilet bowl (see page 37).

How to make a concrete ring beam

A ring beam is a square piece of cast concrete with an open center. It is set into the top of a toilet pit to support the platform and shelter, and to keep the pit walls from collapsing. The ring beam described here can be used along with the platform on page 30 for all pit toilets. Adjust the size of the ring beam to fit the width of the pit.

1. Lay down a plastic sheet or cement bags on level ground.

2. Make a mold of bricks, wooden boards, or both. For a platform that is 120 centimeters by 90 centimeters, the ring beam will be 130 centimeters by 1 meter on the outside, and 1 meter by 70 centimeters on the inside.

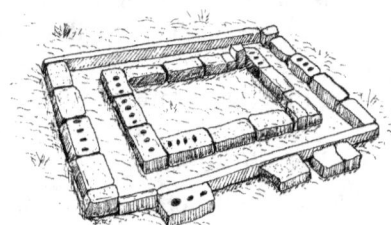

A mold for the ringbeam

3. Make a concrete mix of 1 part cement, 2 parts gravel, 3 parts sand, and enough water so it is wet but holds together. Pour the concrete into the mold until it is half-way to the top.

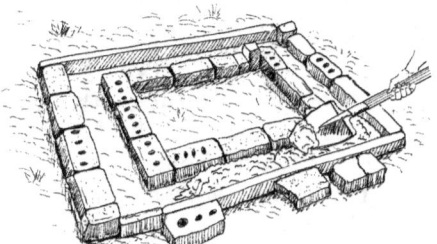

Pouring the concrete

4. Place 2 pieces of reinforcing wire 3 millimeters thick on top of the wet concrete on each side of the ring beam. If you want, you can make handles of wire 8 to 10 millimeters thick, and set them in the concrete near the corners.

5. Pour the rest of the concrete, and smooth it with a block of wood.

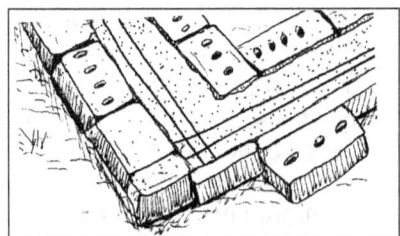

Reinforcing wire

6. Cover the concrete with wet cement sacks, wet cloth, or a plastic sheet and leave it overnight. Wet it several times a day to keep it damp for 7 days.

7. When the ring beam is solid, carry it to the site of the toilet. Level the ground, place the ring beam, and dig a pit inside of it. Pack soil around the outside of the ring beam to set it in place.

8. Place the toilet platform on top, then build a shelter.

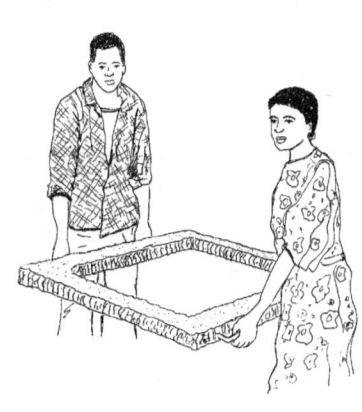

Ventilated improved pit toilets (VIP)

The VIP toilet is a kind of closed pit toilet that reduces smells and flies.

How the VIP works

Wind blows across the top of the vent pipe and carries away smells. The shelter keeps the toilet dark so the flies in the pit will go towards the light at the top of the pipe, get trapped by a wire screen, and die.

To make the VIP toilet

1. Dig the pit 2 meters deep and 1 ½ meters wide. Line the top with bricks or a concrete ring beam sized to fit the pit (see page 31). If the shelter will be very heavy (made of brick, concrete or heavy wood), line the whole pit, except the bottom. Leave gaps in the brick work to let liquids out.

2. Make a platform. See the guidelines on page 30, but make the platform a little bigger: 1 ½ meters by 1 meter, with 2 holes in it. The second hole, at least 11 centimeters wide near an edge of the platform, is for the vent pipe.

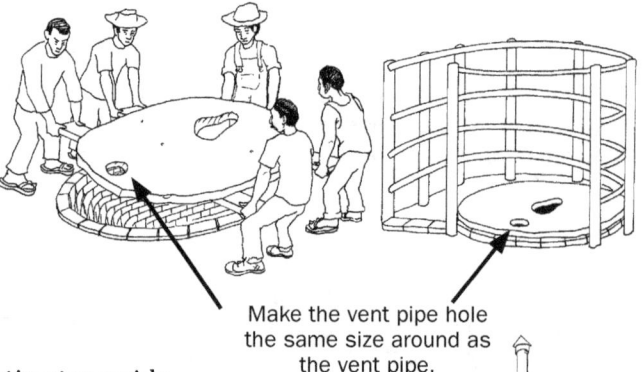

Make the vent pipe hole the same size around as the vent pipe.

3. Build a shelter over the pit and platform.

4. Fit a vent pipe at least 11 centimeters wide into the smaller hole. Paint the vent black to absorb heat and improve ventilation. Cover the top of the vent pipe with a mosquito screen (aluminum or stainless steel last longest) and a 'hat' to protect from rain. Make the vent pipe rise at least 50 centimeters above the roof so the wind can draw out odors.

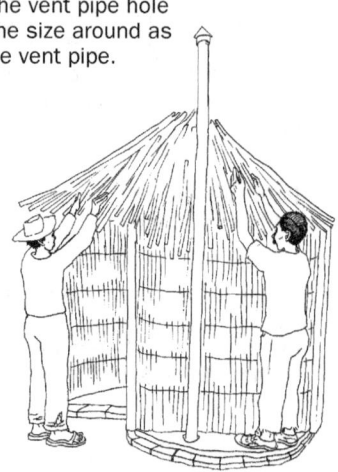

To use and maintain a VIP toilet

Keep the hole covered when not in use. Keep the shelter dark inside. Keep the toilet clean and wash the platform often.

VIP toilets can have these problems

If the shelter is not dark enough, or if the hole is left uncovered, flies will not enter the pipe.

If the vent pipe gets blocked by spider webs, pour water to clean it.

If the shelter has no roof, or if the screen breaks or comes off the vent pipe, there is little fly control.

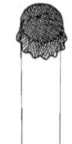

If the wire screen breaks or comes off the pipe, replace it at once.

Ecological toilets

Ecological toilets turn feces and urine into soil conditioner and fertilizer. This improves people's health and the environment by preventing the spread of germs and turning harmful human waste into a valuable resource.

Ecological toilets also protect and conserve water because no water is needed for their use, except for washing. They are safer for groundwater than other toilets because they sit above ground or use shallow pits.

Ecological toilets can be built and used in cities, towns, or villages. They need more maintenance than pit toilets (but not as much as pour-flush toilets), so it is important that people understand how they work.

Turning waste into fertilizer

Rich, healthy soil needs *organic matter* — what is left when plants and other living things die and *decompose*. This natural process of organic matter breaking down into soil is sometimes called *composting*.

Farmers make compost from animal, plant and food waste and add it to the soil. This keeps the soil full of *nutrients* for growing crops. Just as people need nutrients from food to grow strong and healthy, plants need nutrients in soil to grow strong and bear fruit.

The soil grows crops

Fertilizer feeds the soil

Crops become food

Human waste can be turned into fertilizer

Food becomes human waste

Ecological sanitation turns waste into a resource.

Germs and nutrients

Human urine and feces carry nutrients that can improve soil. But feces can also have many germs that cause disease. For this reason, making fertilizer from feces takes more care than composting animal manure and food scraps.

Feces should never be used fresh. But once made into fertilizer, feces can safely help grow food, trees, and other crops without chemical fertilizers.

Urine carries fewer germs than feces and has more nutrients. This makes it safer to handle and very valuable as fertilizer. But urine is too strong to use directly on plants, so it also needs special treatment (see pages 41-42).

Compost toilets and urine-diverting dry toilets

There are 2 main types of ecological toilets: 'compost toilets' and 'urine-diverting' or 'dry' toilets. Both kinds can create safe fertilizer. Many people call both kinds 'compost toilets.' But there are some important differences.

In compost toilets:

- Feces and urine go into a container that will not leak into the groundwater, like a shallow pit or a large concrete box.

- The user adds a mix of dry matter such as straw, leaves, sawdust, and soil after each use. This reduces smells and helps the waste to break down and become compost.

- Excrement is stored until it heats up and breaks down. The mix will heat up and kill most germs, including roundworm eggs (the hardest to kill). To heat up well, it must be slightly damp.

- After the mix has had a long time to kill germs (usually 1 year), the dry matter is removed for use as fertilizer.

In dry toilets:

- Urine is kept separate from feces. It is collected, processed, and used as fertilizer.

- Feces go into a container, like a large concrete box or a hard plastic movable container that will not leak into groundwater.

- The user adds soil mixed with dry plant matter and ash to the feces after each use. This reduces smells and helps the waste to dry out.

- The feces never get mixed with water. A dry mix will kill most germs, including roundworm eggs.

- The feces is stored for up to 1 year, until it has the texture of dry soil.

For both of these toilets, the aged feces mixture is ready after 1 year to be mixed into a compost pile, emptied into a shallow pit for planting a tree, or added directly into the soil for planting.

Dry toilets help local economy

In several towns in Morelos, Mexico, many people use ecological dry toilets. One neighborhood called La Cienega, or The Swamp, has a special need for dry toilets. Because the neighborhood is in a wet, lowland area, pit toilets do not work. To solve the problem, members of the community bought a special kind of toilet bowl that separates urine from feces. These toilet bowls are built locally in small workshops that support several workers. The workers train community groups how to use these new toilet bowls.

Many people in La Cienega make a living by growing and selling fruit trees and other plants. The first people in the neighborhood to use dry toilets discovered that they could use the urine and compost from their toilets as fertilizer for the trees. When their neighbors saw the trees grow big and healthy, they too wanted to try these new toilets that give free fertilizer.

Now almost every family in La Cienega uses these toilets. The local workshop is busy making them, and the community has grown both healthier and wealthier.

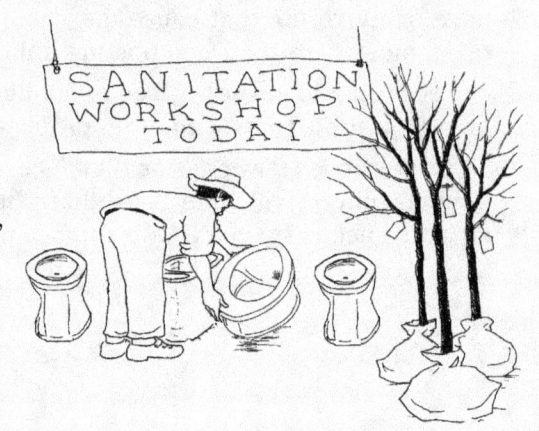

Simple compost toilet for tree planting

This toilet makes fertilizer for planting trees. It is simple to build, and is made so the shelter can be moved when the pit is full.

This toilet is best where there is space and a desire to plant trees. It is also good for places with high groundwater, because the pit is shallow. Covering the toilet pit with soil and planting a tree there helps to decompose the waste.

This is a great way to start an orchard of fruit trees or other useful trees. If you do not plan to plant trees, use a different type of toilet.

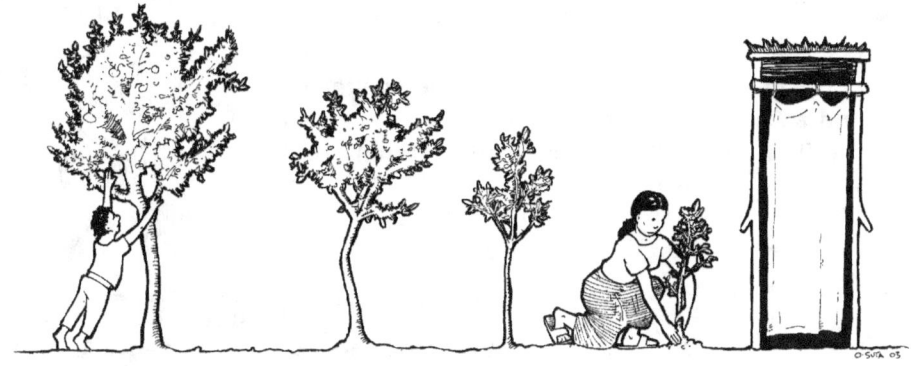

To build a simple toilet for tree planting

Level the ground and place a concrete ring beam (see page 33) where you want the toilet. Inside the ring beam, dig a pit 1 meter deep, and secure the ring beam in place. Make a platform to put over the pit and ring beam. Build a light shelter that will be easy to move.

To use and maintain this toilet

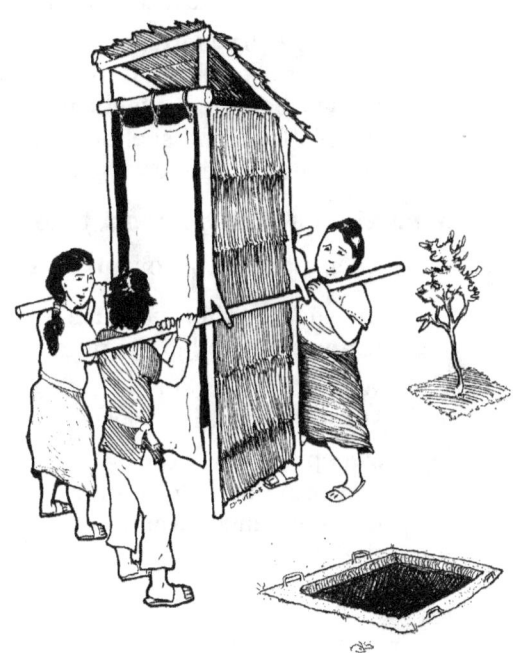

- Before using, put dry leaves or straw in the pit. This will help feces decompose.
- Add a handful of soil mixed with ashes or dry leaves after every use.
- When the pile gets too high, stir it down with a stick.
- Sweep and wash the platform often. Be careful not to get much water in the pit.
- When the hole is nearly full, remove the shelter, platform, and ring beam.
- Fill the hole with 15 centimeters of soil mixed with plant matter. After several weeks, the waste will settle. Add more soil and plant matter, water, and plant a tree. Fruit trees grow well and bear safe and abundant fruit.
- Move the shelter, platform, and ring beam. Dig another hole, and do it again.

2-pit compost toilet

The 2-pit compost toilet is like the simple compost toilet for treeplanting, but rather than planting a tree in the pit, the compost is dug out and used in the garden or fields. This toilet tends to be safer for groundwater than traditional pit toilets because the waste is mixed with soil in a shallow pit, allowed to dry out and kill germs, and then removed.

To build a 2 pit compost toilet

Dig 2 pits 1 to 1 ½ meters deep, 1 meter wide, and 30 centimeters apart. Add a lining or ring beam to both pits (see page 31). Place a platform and a simple shelter over one pit, and a concrete or wood cover over the second pit. Use the first pit until it is nearly full. A family of 6 will fill the pit in about 1 year.

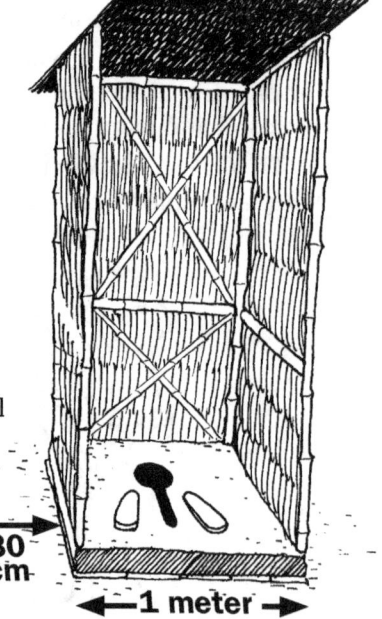

1. When the first pit is almost full, fill it with 30 centimeters of soil and cover it with a board or concrete slab. Move the platform and shelter to the other pit, and use it until it is nearly full. Leave the first pit alone – or, after it has settled for 2 months, add more soil and plant a seasonal vegetable like tomatoes right in the pit. Since the feces are still being processed, it is best to avoid root crops that grow underground, such as carrots and potatoes.

2. When the second pit is full, empty the first pit with a shovel. Wear gloves, and wash hands after handling the fresh fertilizer.

3. Store the dry matter from the pit in open bags or buckets for later use, or add it to a compost pile or garden. (To know when the contents are ready, see page 41.) Move the platform and shelter back to the first pit, while the contents of the second pit settle. And so on...

To maintain a 2 pit compost toilet

*   Keep a bucket of soil mixed with dry plant matter in the shelter. After each use, throw a handful in the pit.

*   When the pile gets too high, stir it down with a stick.

*   Sweep and wash the platform often. Be careful not to get much water in the pit.

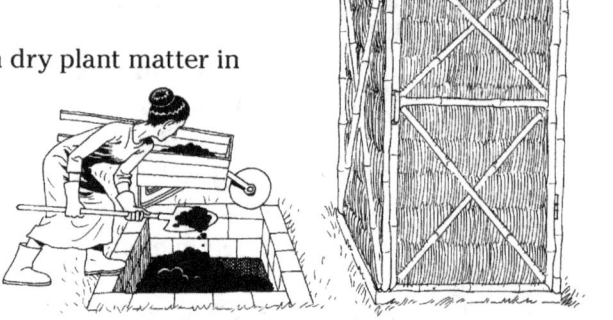

After 1 year the contents of the 2 pit compost toilet should be safe to mix into garden soil as fertilizer. But it is still best to wear gloves and shoes when handling it.

Urine-diverting dry toilets

Dry toilets do not use pits. They are built above ground, so it is easier to remove the contents. They also have a toilet bowl with separate compartments that keep urine and feces apart. This helps the contents of the toilet stay dry, which kills germs and reduces smells. This also allows the urine to be used as fertilizer. Because they are built above ground and lined on the bottom, they are safe for groundwater.

Dry toilets are more costly to build than pit toilets. Their safe use requires training, because they are used differently than pit toilets and water-based toilets. And it takes some work to keep them well maintained. But they are very good for people who want to produce fertilizer from their wastes. They are also a good choice in places where:

- The groundwater is too high for pit toilets.
- Flooding is common.
- The ground is too hard to dig.
- People want a permanent toilet in or near their house.

2 chamber dry toilets

This dry toilet has 2 chambers where feces break down into safe fertilizer. One side is used as the toilet while the feces on the other side dry and break down. A special toilet bowl that works for both men and women separates urine from feces. The urine drains through a hose into a container outside of the toilet. After about a year, the dried feces are removed and added to a compost pile or used on fields or gardens. The collected urine can be mixed with water and used as fertilizer (see pages 41 to 42).

Parts of the 2 chamber dry toilet

Shelter for comfort, privacy, and to keep the toilet dry.

Front of toilet

Back of toilet

Hose to divert urine from urinal and bowl to urine pot.

Urine pot where the urine is collected from the toilet and the urinal.

Urinal

2 chambers made of brick, concrete, or other waterproof material. While one is in use as a toilet, feces dry and decompose in the other.

One kind of dry toilet uses a **toilet bowl** that separates urine from feces. The bowl looks very much like any toilet bowl, but it does not use water. Home-made urine catching devices can work just as well (see pages 38-39).

Small doors at the back where the dried feces can be removed.

3 ways to build a dry toilet

All 3 have a base made of concrete, brick, or any other waterproof material with these parts:

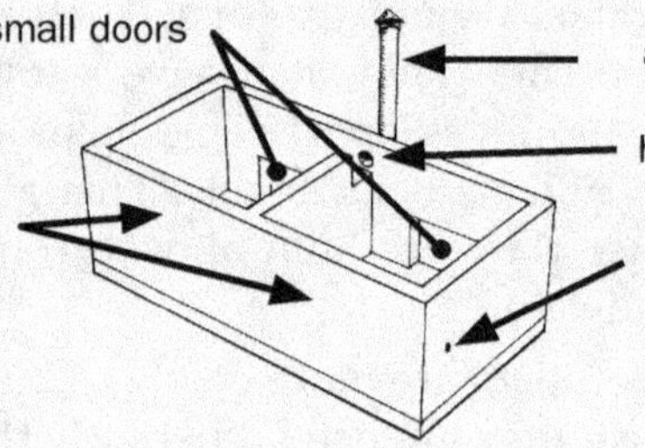

2 small doors

2 chambers

a vent pipe

hole for vent pipe

a hole on each side or in the front for the urine-diverting hose to run out of the chamber

Types of toilets	*Building the base*	*How the urine is separated*
For squatting 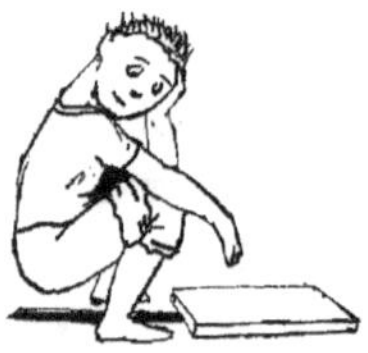 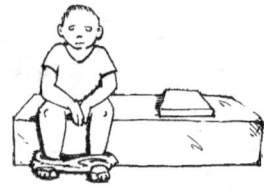	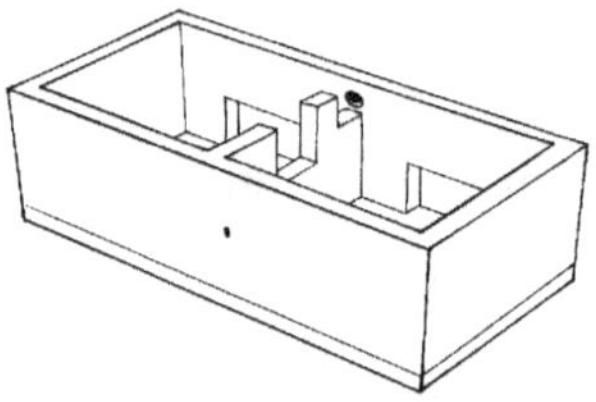 Leave a space in the dividing wall for a urine-separating container to serve both chambers.	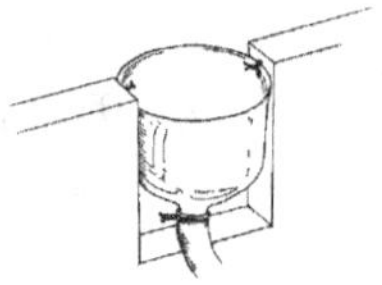 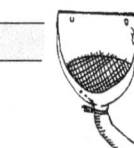 Cut the bottom off a 20 liter jug. Attach it, upside-down, to the space in the wall dividing both chambers. Attach a tube to the spout to divert urine, making sure there are no leaks between the jug and the tube. Put a fine mesh screen in the jug to keep feces and other things from falling in.
For sitting, with a bench	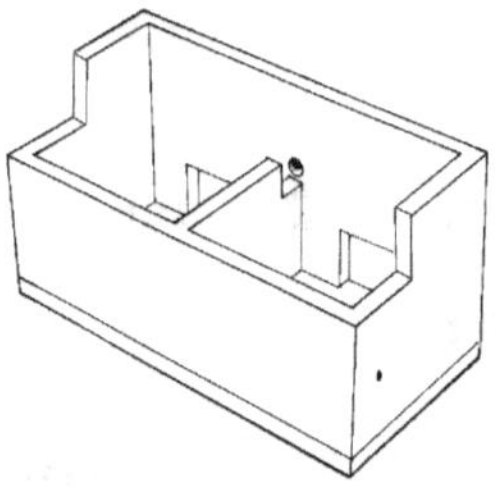 Build the back of the base up to make a bench across both chambers.	Cut the bottom and side from a plastic jug. Attach a tube to the spout to divert urine. Put a fine mesh screen in the jug to keep feces and other things from falling in.
For sitting, with a toilet bowl 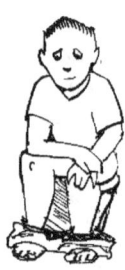	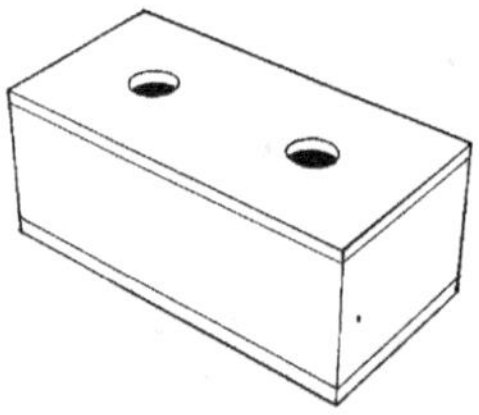 Cover the base with a level platform of wood or concrete with a hole over each chamber.	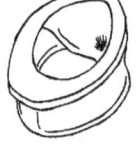 Urine-diverting toilet bowls can be built or bought in some places. If they are available, they are very easy to install and use.

3 ways to build a dry toilet

For all 3, build a shelter and steps. Attach doors in the back (cement slabs held in place by lime mortar work well). Run the urine-diverting tube out the hole in the toilet base to a container, a drainage pit, or into the garden to fertilize the soil.

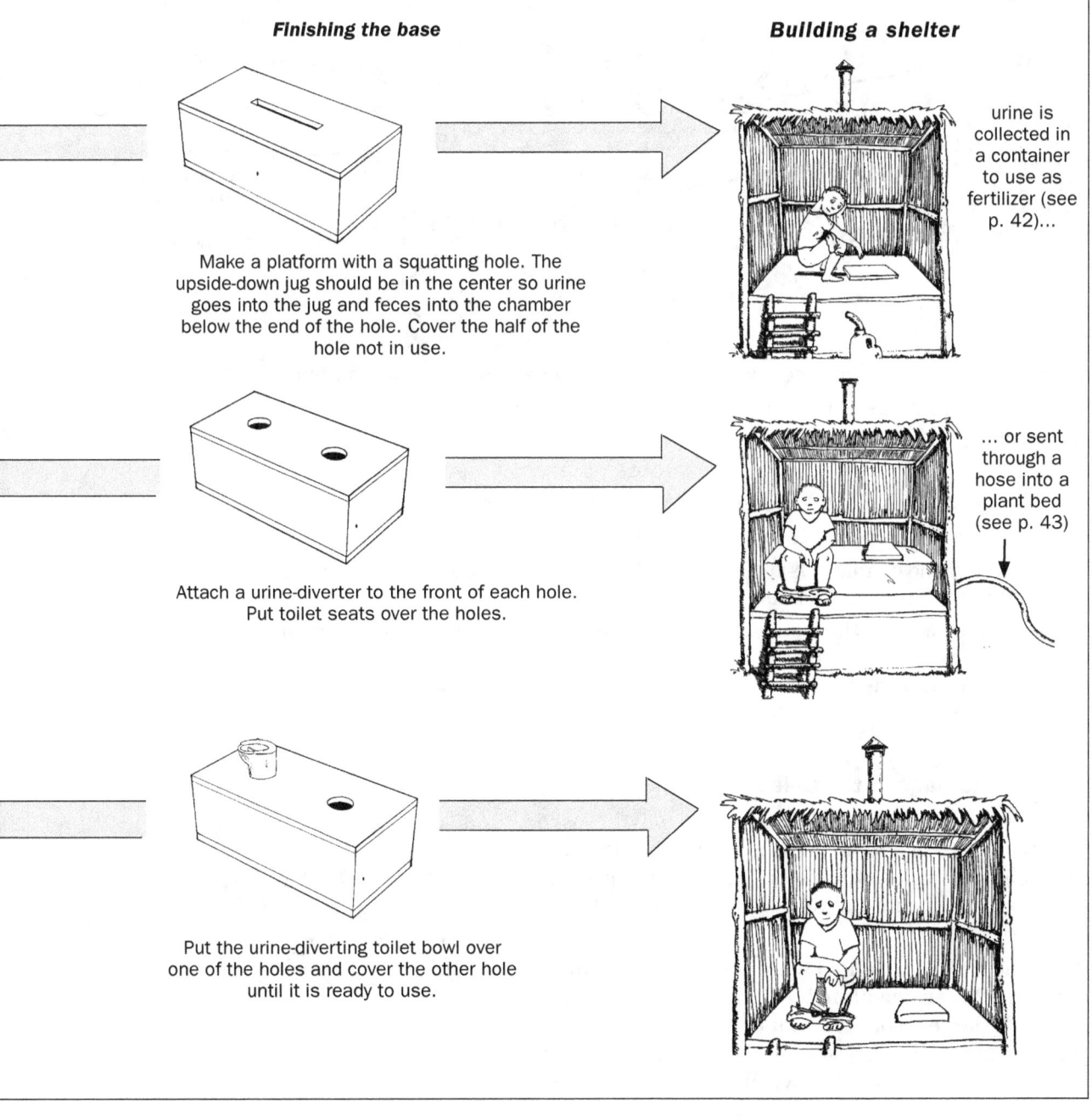

Finishing the base

Make a platform with a squatting hole. The upside-down jug should be in the center so urine goes into the jug and feces into the chamber below the end of the hole. Cover the half of the hole not in use.

Attach a urine-diverter to the front of each hole. Put toilet seats over the holes.

Put the urine-diverting toilet bowl over one of the holes and cover the other hole until it is ready to use.

Building a shelter

urine is collected in a container to use as fertilizer (see p. 42)...

... or sent through a hose into a plant bed (see p. 43)

To use and maintain a 2 chamber dry toilet

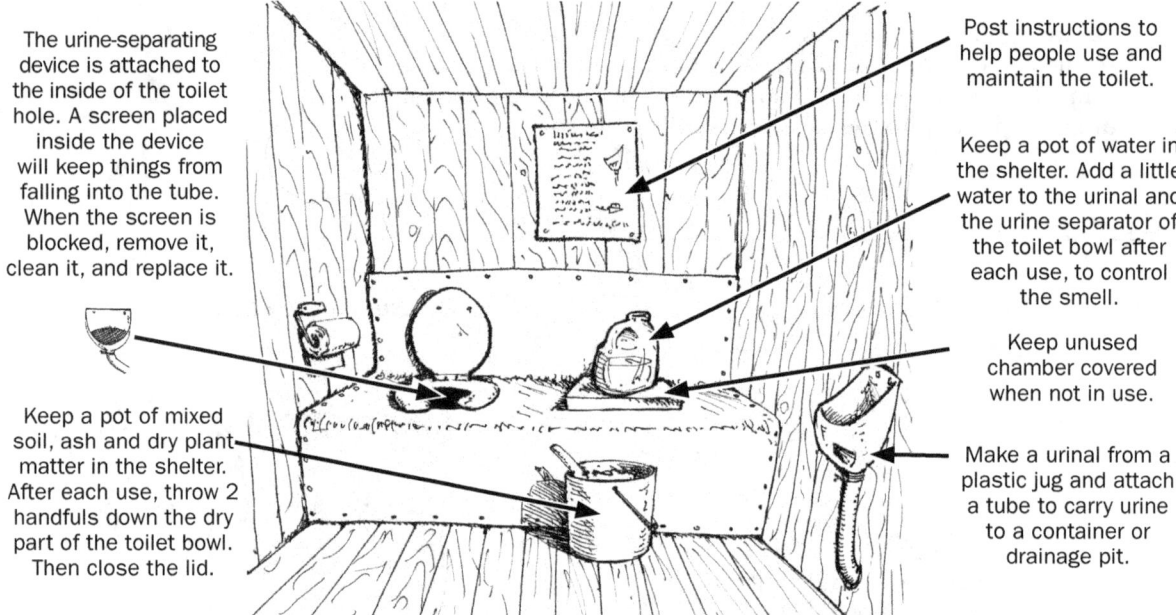

The urine-separating device is attached to the inside of the toilet hole. A screen placed inside the device will keep things from falling into the tube. When the screen is blocked, remove it, clean it, and replace it.

Keep a pot of mixed soil, ash and dry plant matter in the shelter. After each use, throw 2 handfuls down the dry part of the toilet bowl. Then close the lid.

Post instructions to help people use and maintain the toilet.

Keep a pot of water in the shelter. Add a little water to the urinal and the urine separator of the toilet bowl after each use, to control the smell.

Keep unused chamber covered when not in use.

Make a urinal from a plastic jug and attach a tube to carry urine to a container or drainage pit.

- Make sure no water gets in the feces holding part of the toilet chamber.
- If the contents of the toilet get wet, add more dry matter.
- If the toilet smells bad, add more dry matter and make sure the vent pipe is clear.
- If the pile builds up too high, use a stick to push it back down.
- When the urine pot is full, empty it and make fertilizer. (See pages 41 to 42.)
- When one chamber is full, use the other chamber. Be sure to cover the chamber that is not being used.
- It is best to let the feces sit for a full year before emptying the chamber. After a year, or when the second chamber is full, empty the first chamber and repeat the process.

Do not put garbage in the toilet

For ecological toilets to work, they must only be used for excrement. Women having their monthly bleeding may safely use ecological toilets. But sanitary pads and other products should be put in trash bins – not in the toilet.

Ecological toilets cannot be used to dispose of things that will not break down, such as cans, bottles, plastic, tampons, or large amounts of paper. It is OK to use small amounts of paper, leaves, sawdust and other plant matter because these things break down and can be turned back into the soil.

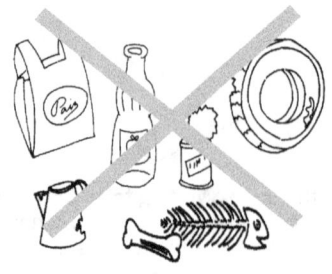

Do not put garbage in the toilet.

To know when the solid fertilizer is safe for use

The contents of a dry toilet are ready to remove when they are dry, and have little or no smell. For this to happen, they should be kept dry inside the toilet chamber for 1 year.

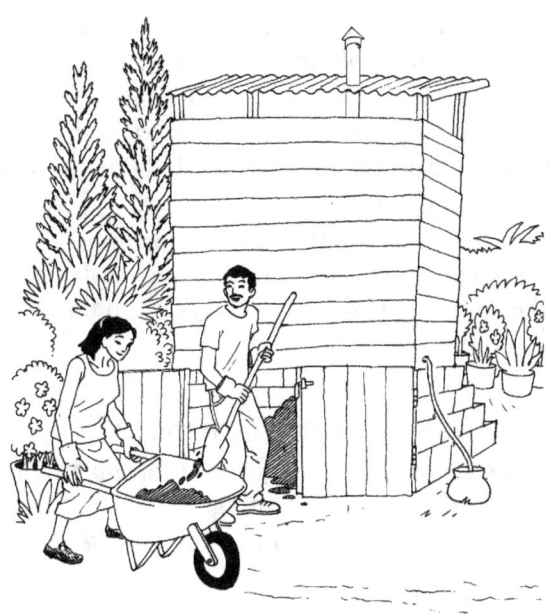

Remove dry material for use as fertilizer.

When you think the contents are ready to remove, open the chamber. If the pile is wet, add dry plant matter or soil mixed with ash and let it sit for several more weeks. If the pile is dry and does not have a strong smell, it is ready. Remove it with a shovel.

After drying out for 1 year, most germs will be dead and the material should be safe to handle and to add directly to garden soil. But if there is any doubt, the contents of the toilet can be given extra treatment to ensure that all germs are killed. To completely dry the contents of the toilet, store it in bags or buckets for a few weeks. To heat it up, leave it in a dry, sunny area, or add it to a compost pile.

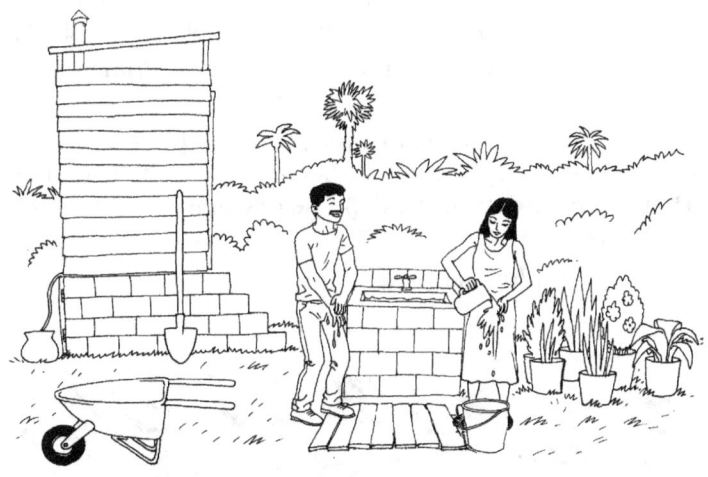

Wear gloves and shoes when handling human waste and always wash after emptying the toilet.

Urine fertilizer

Some farmers use urine mixed with water as a fertilizer because urine carries valuable nutrients like nitrogen and phosphorous that can help plants grow. Urine is much safer to handle than feces. However, the same nutrients that make it a good fertilizer can pollute water sources. Also, urine can carry blood-flukes (schistosomiasis) -- common in only some parts of the world. Because of this, it is important not to put urine into water sources, or near where people drink or bathe.

To make simple urine fertilizer

Store urine for a few days in a closed container. This will kill any germs the urine contains, and will also prevent nutrients from escaping into the air.

To make fertilizer, *dilute* the urine with water — mix 3 containers of water for every 1 of urine. (Undiluted, fresh urine is too strong and may damage plants.) You can fertilize plants with diluted urine as often as 3 times a week.

Plants fertilized with urine can grow as well as plants grown with chemical fertilizers, and need less water. Plants that make edible leaves, like spinach, grow best. Always wash hands after handling urine.

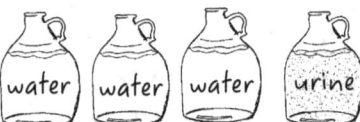

3 jugs of water plus 1 jug of urine = safe fertilizer

To make fermented urine fertilizer

Adding compost to urine, and letting this mixture *ferment* (rot and turn sour), can create new soil for planting.

1. Collect urine from dry toilets. For each liter of urine, add 1 tablespoon of rich soil or compost.

2. Let the mix sit uncovered for 4 weeks. This will smell bad, so do it in a place away from people. The urine mixture will ferment and turn brown.

3. Fill a large container with dry leaves, straw, or other dry plant matter. Line the container with thick plastic to prevent water leakage through the hole in the bottom.

4. Add fermented urine. The best mix is 7 parts plant matter to 1 part urine (about 3 liters of urine for every 30 cubic centimeters of plant matter.)

5. Cover with a thin layer of soil – no more than 10 centimeters. Plant seeds or seedlings.

6. Water every 2 days with a mix of 1 part urine to 10 parts water. (This is a weaker mix than we suggest above, because it will be used in closed containers rather than open gardens or fields.) The dry plant matter will turn to rich soil in 10 to 12 months.

The new soil can be used for planting.

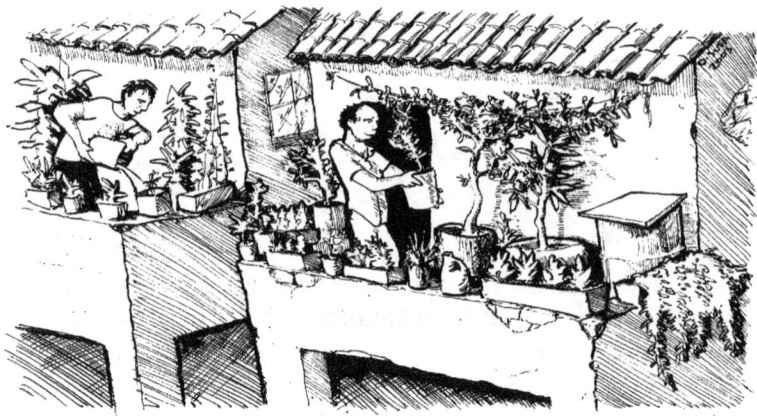

Urban gardening with urine fertilizer

Improved and adapted dry toilets

The toilets in this book are only some of the options for ecological sanitation. They can be improved and adapted to meet the needs of different communities. Some things that will make a dry toilet work better are:

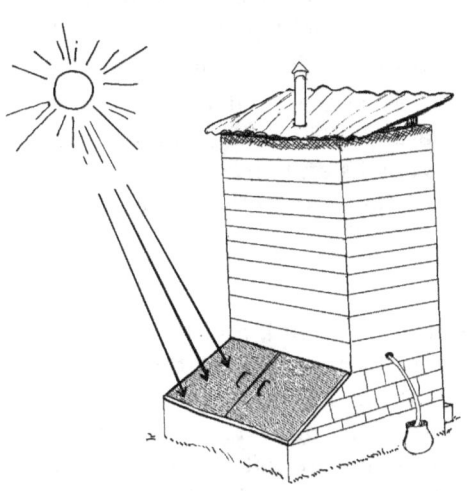

Heat from the sun

Build the toilet so that the chamber doors face the sun, and paint the door panels black. This will make the chambers heat up, improve ventilation, and kill germs faster.

More air flow

Laying bamboo, corn stalks, branches, or other dry plant matter on the floor of the chamber before use will help air flow through the feces for faster drying.

A wash toilet with plant bed

People in India have adapted the dry toilet to let both urine and wash water drain into a bed of reeds.

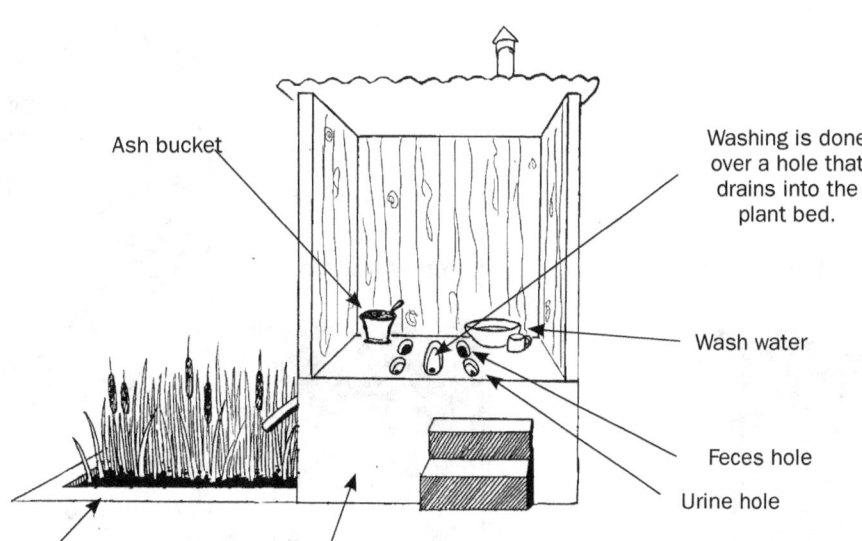

Ash bucket

Washing is done over a hole that drains into the plant bed.

Wash water

Feces hole

Urine hole

The plant bed where the wash water and urine go is filled with sand and gravel and planted with reeds or other local, non-edible plants. When the plants grow too big, they are cut back and thrown into the toilet.

The chambers under the toilet are lined with straw before use, to absorb moisture and make a good bed for the compost. Every time it is used, 1 or 2 handfuls of soil or ash are thrown in. Every now and then, some dry plant matter is added to help the material dry and decompose. After one year of use, the first chamber is opened and the material is put in a compost pile or dug into the soil for planting.

Pour-flush pit toilets

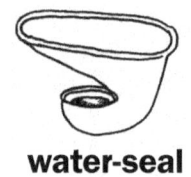

water-seal trap

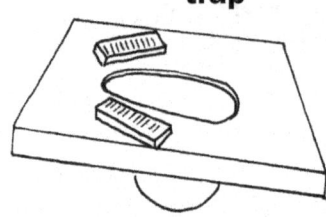

water-seal trap set in concrete platform

Pour-flush toilets use water to flush waste into a pit. These toilets are common in both urban and rural areas where water is used to clean the anus after defecating. They are not much more costly than pit toilets. Because well-built pour-flush toilets prevent smells, they can be built in or near the home.

Pour-flush toilets use a plastic, fiberglass, or cement bowl or squatting pan set into a concrete platform. The bowl or pan often has a 'water-seal trap' that prevents smells and insect breeding in the wet pits. The concrete platform is placed directly over a pit. Or it can be connected by pipe to a pit or 2 pits.

How to use a pour-flush toilet

When there is 1 pit, the toilet is used until full, and then it must be emptied before it can continue to be used. When there are 2 pits, there is a junction box that directs waste towards the pit in use. The first pit is used until near full. Then waste is diverted into the second pit. Its contents are left to settle for at least 2 years, until it can be emptied without risk of illness from germs. The second pit is used until the first pit is emptied, and then it is allowed to settle as the first pit is used again.

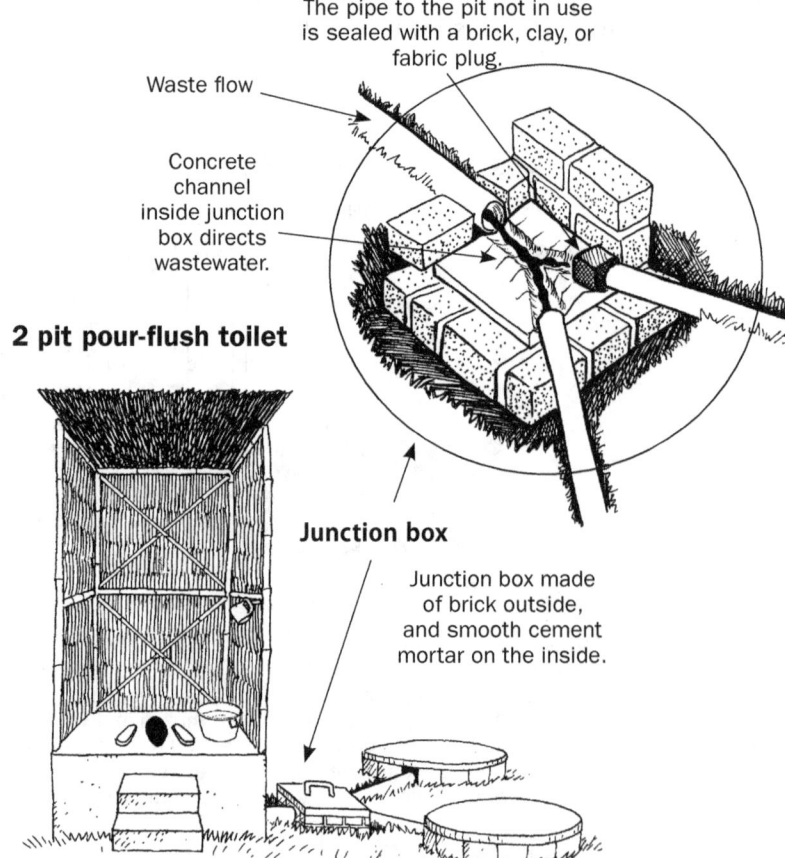

The pipe to the pit not in use is sealed with a brick, clay, or fabric plug.

Waste flow

Concrete channel inside junction box directs wastewater.

Junction box

Junction box made of brick outside, and smooth cement mortar on the inside.

1 pit pour-flush toilet

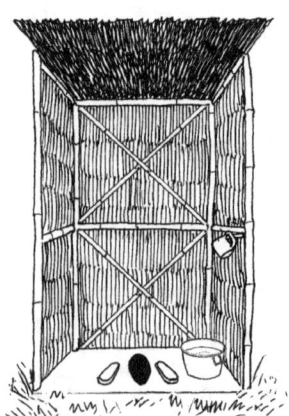

One lined pit underground, 2 meters deep. A family of 5 will fill this pit in about 5 years time.

2 pit pour-flush toilet

Above ground chamber allows wastewater to flow down to pits. With regular care, this toilet will last many, many years.

What to know when building a 2 pit pour-flush toilet

Depending on soil conditions and groundwater level, pour-flush toilets should never be built less than 3 meters from wells. In wet soil conditions the toilets should be at least 20 meters from wells.

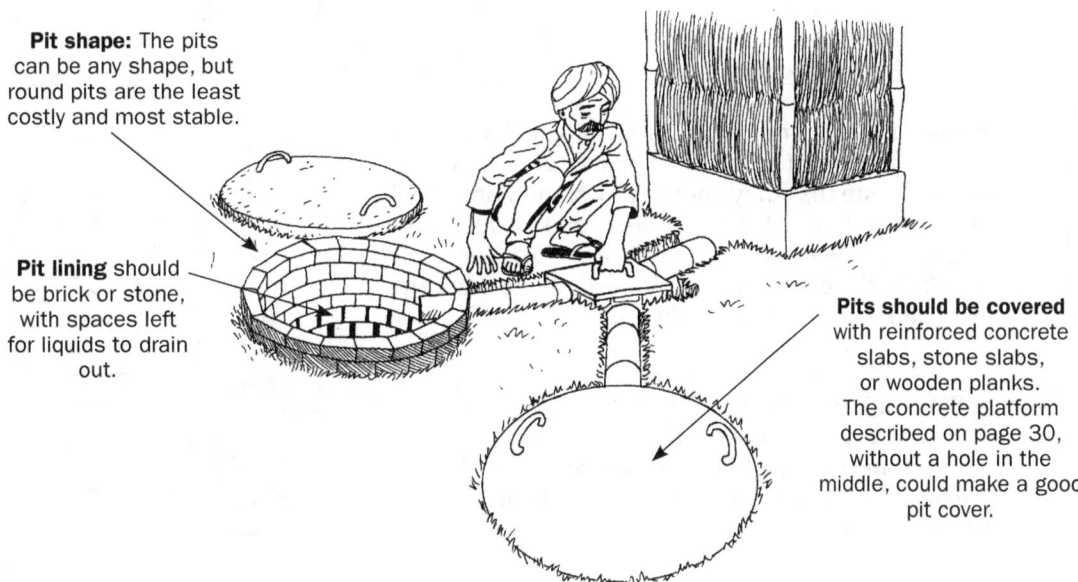

Pit shape: The pits can be any shape, but round pits are the least costly and most stable.

Pit lining should be brick or stone, with spaces left for liquids to drain out.

Pits should be covered with reinforced concrete slabs, stone slabs, or wooden planks. The concrete platform described on page 30, without a hole in the middle, could make a good pit cover.

To use and maintain a pour-flush toilet

Water must be poured in after every use. Pouring a little water in before using will also help keep the pan clean.

Clean the toilet daily. To clean the squatting pan, use detergent powder and a long-handled brush. The pits can overflow if:

- the water seal gets blocked. If this happens, the toilet will not work.
- the groundwater is less than 3 meters deep. If this is true, there is a risk of groundwater contamination.

Emptying the pit

After about 3 years of use the first pit will be full. Divert the waste into the second pit, while the first pit rests. If soil conditions and moisture are favorable, the waste will slowly and safely absorb into the soil and the pit will not need emptying.

Remove the pit cover, add a layer of soil about 30 centimeters (2 hands-widths) deep, and replace the cover. After 2 years, the contents can be removed with a shovel and used as fertilizer.

SANITATION STEPS TO HEALTHY COMMUNITIES

No toilet is right for all situations and each sanitation method has room for improvement. This activity helps people think about what toilets are available and decide which one is best for them.

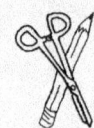

Time: 1 to 2 hours

Materials: small drawing paper, large drawing paper, colored pens or markers, sticky tape.

➡ **Step 1:** Make groups of 5 or so people. Each person draws a picture of every toilet or way of disposing of human waste that they know. They should draw their own toilets, others they have seen, and even pictures of what people do where there is no toilet. The goal is to have the group draw a range of toilets, from the most simple to the most modern.

➡ **Step 2:** When the pictures are ready, each small group arranges their pictures in order, from what they think are the worst to the best. These are taped to large sheets of paper.

➡ **Step 3:** Each group shows its pictures and tells the reason for the order they chose. What makes one system better and another worse? Each group member also tells which toilet he or she uses at home – and which he or she would like to have.

➡ **Step 4:** After everyone has shown their drawings, the group talks about the difference between all methods.

Ask questions like:
- Does everyone agree about which toilet is worst and which is best?
- Is there one toilet that seems best to everyone? Why?
- Are there some toilets that no one in the group uses? Why?

This can lead to a discussion of the reasons for people's choices.
- What health benefits are most important?
- What environmental benefits are most important?
- Which toilet would people prefer? Is this because of health reasons, cost, or for some other reason?
- Would any of the improvements people want require changes in local conditions or how people think about sanitation? Are there simple things that can be done to improve what already exists?
- If the group includes both men and women, are their answers different?

SANITATION STEPS TO HEALTHY COMMUNITIES

➡ **Step 5:** Introduce other toilets that people may not know about. This may include small changes to their current toilets such as vent pipes, or new options such as ecological toilets. (It may include all the toilets in this book, and others you may know of.) The group discusses these new ideas.

> To know what changes are needed, decide what health benefits and environmental benefits matter most.

> To know what changes are possible, decide which sanitation systems people want and can afford.

➡ **Step 6:** Lead a discussion about the different methods, asking the group to think about questions in the chart below. Each person shares his or her opinion about the benefits and risks of each toilet, using numbers to show how strongly he or she feels. For example, 5 may mean the best and 0 may mean the worst. Mark each person's opinion on the chart and count to see which method is judged best.

	Health benefits?	Environmental benefits?	Cost?	Work to clean and maintain
No toilet				
Closed pit toilet				
VIP toilet				
Compost toilet				
Dry toilet				

➡ **Step 7:** The group makes new drawings based on the discussion of benefits and the new methods they have learned about. They tape the new and old drawings to large sheets of paper in order from best to worst. Finally, they compare the new order of the method to the earlier order they had chosen.

- What differences are there?
- What ideas or information caused people to change their minds about what toilets are worst and best?

Based on this discussion, the group can decide what toilet or improvement is best for them.

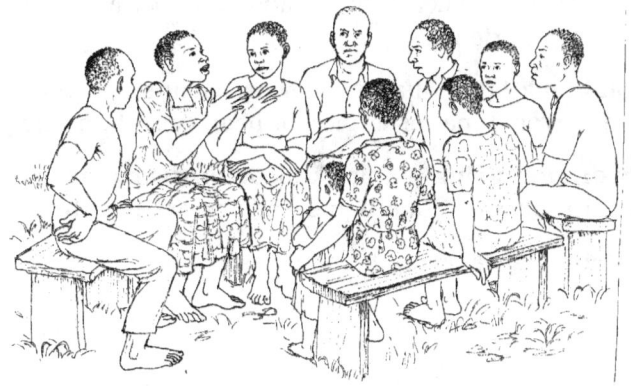

Communication among men and women is an important part of choosing safe and healthy toilets.

Vocabulary

Compost – plant matter and manure that has broken down and turned into fertilizer. To work well, composting (the process of making compost) requires a mix of different elements, such as dry plant matter, wet plant matter, other nutrients, air and moisture.

Decompose – when living things are broken down by heat, insects, and bacteria. When plant matter decomposes, it turns to compost or rich soil.

Dehydration – loss of fluid. Dehydration is one sign of diarrhea diseases related to unhealthy sanitation. Dehydration can be very dangerous, especially for children.

Dilute – make weaker by mixing with water.

Ecological – imitating or acting like a natural system. Sanitation can be called ecological when it recycles nutrients by returning them to the earth. Compost toilets and dry toilets are ecological.

Ferment – when food or other organic matter rots and becomes sour. This happens because bacteria enter and change the nature of the substance. Compost can also be said to be fermenting.

Germs – tiny living things that can spread disease. Different germs cause different health problems and spread in different ways. For example, dysentery germs are spread through feces, tuberculosis germs spread through the air, and scabies spreads through clothes and bedding.

Groundwater – water that flows underground. Groundwater is the source of drinking water in wells and springs. Groundwater may also be called a water table or an aquifer. The groundwater level changes depending on rainfall and water use.

Hygiene – things people do to stay clean and prevent the spread of germs. Hygiene includes washing hands and bathing, storing and preparing food, and keeping the home clean.

Nutrient – anything that feeds plants, animals, or people. People need nutrients in food to grow strong and healthy, and plants need nutrients in soil to grow strong and bear fruit. When farmers add compost and fertilizer to the soil, these are ways of adding nutrients.

Organic matter – what is left when plants and other living things die and break down. Organic matter is part of healthy soil and helps plants grow.

Rehydration drink – a drink made of sugar, salt, and water or from grain and water that helps retain liquid and restore health when a person is dehydrated.

Sanitation – managing human waste in a safe and healthy way.

www.ingramcontent.com/pod-product-compliance
Lightning Source LLC
Chambersburg PA
CBHW080900170526
45158CB00009B/2784